Table of Contents

PART ONE
WHY ARE CATASTROPHIC AND LONG-TERM HEALTH CARE PUBLIC POLICY ISSUES?

PART TWO
A SEARCH FOR DEFINITIONS AND SOLUTIONS

1989

Where Coverage Ends:

Catastrophic Illness and Long-Term Health Care Costs

AN EBRI-ERF
POLICY FORUM

EBRI

**EMPLOYEE BENEFIT
RESEARCH INSTITUTE**

© 1988 Employee Benefit Research Institute
Education and Research Fund
2121 K Street, NW, Suite 600
Washington, DC 20037-2121
(202) 659-0670

Library of Congress Cataloging in Publication Data

EBRI-ERF 18th Policy Forum (1987: Washington, D.C.)
    Where coverage ends: catastrophic illness and long-term health care costs an EBRI-ERF Policy Forum.
        p. cm.
    "Dallas L. Salisbury"—CIP foreword.
    The forum was held October 21, 1987 in Washington, D.C.
    Includes index.
    ISBN 0-86643-061-X
    1. Insurance, Health—Government policy—United States—Congresses.
    2. Insurance, Long-term care—United States—Congresses.   3. Medical care, Cost of—United States—Congresses.   I. Salisbury, Dallas L.   II. Employee Benefit Research Institute (Washington, D.C.). Education and Research Fund.
    III. Title.
HD7102.U4E27   1987
368.3'8'00973—dc19   88-16237
                                                                                    CIP

Printed in the United States of America

PART THREE
APPROACHES TO INSURANCE

PART FOUR
PUBLIC AND PRIVATE ROLES IN CATASTROPHIC AND LONG-TERM CARE

PART FIVE
WHAT DOES THE FUTURE HOLD?

List of Tables and Charts

Chart

Foreword

Catastrophic medical expenses are usually associated with the older members of society, but they can affect individuals in any age group. Whether they occur as a consequence of lengthy hospitalization, high cost medical procedures, or the need for long-term care at home or in a skilled nursing facility, these expenses can bring financial devastation to individuals and families if they have not planned carefully. Most Americans have not.

Current forms of insurance—private and public, including Medicare and Medicaid—provide adequately for these events for some, but not for most. Many health care expenses are not fully covered under private insurance or, as a means of managing use, require high copayments by individuals. Medicaid offers financial support, but only after an individual has exhausted most of his or her resources. And for many individuals without health insurance, any major illness can result in a catastrophic level of expense.

The role of government, employers, and the individual in protecting against catastrophic medical expense has been debated for decades, but 1987 saw the focusing of that debate with a major catastrophic health care financing proposal introduced by the Reagan administration. The debate was also a prominent part of the 1988 presidential campaign.

On October 21, 1987, the Employee Benefit Research Institute's Education and Research Fund sponsored a policy forum to discuss issues and proposals related to catastrophic expenses. The forum brought together corporate executives, government officials, and representatives from labor, academia, elderly and research organizations.

Where Coverage Ends: Catastrophic Illness and Long-Term Health Care Costs integrates the papers and proceedings of the policy forum into a single work, organized into five parts. The book's chapters examine present catastrophic and long-term health care policy, various definitions of catastrophic expenses, the level of need, public- and private-sector roles, and a view of the future.

On behalf of EBRI and its Education and Research Fund, I wish to thank the policy forum speakers and participants for their substantial contributions to this book. We believe it will assist policymakers, benefit experts, and the public in better understanding what the catastrophic and long-term health care debates are about: the background and the issues, the arguments for and against an expansion of the government role, and the impact on the economy of alternative initiatives. Special thanks are due to Frank McArdle and Nancy Newman for planning the policy forum, to Barbara Coleman and Deborah Holmes for compiling, editing, and producing this book, and to Christine Dolan for creating the index.

The views expressed in this book are solely those of the authors and the forum participants. They should not be attributed to the officers, trustees, members, or associates of EBRI, its staff or its Education and Research Fund.

DALLAS L. SALISBURY
President
Employee Benefit Research Institute

July 1988

About the Authors

ROBERT M. BALL

Mr. Ball is a consultant on social security, health, and welfare policy. Ball served as U.S. Commissioner of Social Security under presidents Kennedy, Johnson, and Nixon. He was also a member of the 1979 statutory Advisory Council on Social Security and the President's National Commission on Social Security Reform, which made recommendations leading to the 1983 amendments to the Social Security Act. From 1973 to 1981, Ball was a senior scholar at the Institute of Medicine, National Academy of Sciences.

CHARLES BETLEY

Mr. Betley is a research assistant at the Employee Benefit Research Institute (EBRI), where he has worked on long-term care, retiree health, and other issues of health care financing and service delivery. Before joining EBRI, Betley was with the U.S. Congress Office of Technology Assessment, where he worked on a study evaluating alternative methods of paying for physicians' services under Medicare. He received a bachelor's degree in Public Policy Studies from Duke University in 1984, and has done graduate work in economics at George Washington University.

DEBORAH J. CHOLLET

Dr. Chollet is senior research associate at the Employee Benefit Research Institute, where she conducts research on private health insurance and public health care financing. Prior to joining EBRI, Dr. Chollet was a senior research fellow at the National Center for Health Services Research, U.S. Department of Health and Human Services and served on the economics faculty of Temple University.

Dr. Chollet holds a master's and doctorate in economics at the Maxwell School of Citizenship and Public Affairs, Syracuse University. She has written and lectured extensively in the areas of private and public health insurance programs, medical malpractice insurance, and private employee benefit plans.

ROBERT B. FRIEDLAND

Dr. Friedland is a research associate at the Employee Benefit Research Institute. Before joining EBRI, he was senior economist for Maryland's medical care programs, Department of Health and Mental Hygiene; assistant professor of economics in the School of Business and Economics at Towson State University; and a fellow at the National Institute on Aging. Friedland is directing EBRI's policy study on financing long-term care.

MARY JO GIBSON

Ms. Gibson is a health policy analyst in the Public Policy Institute at the American Association of Retired Persons. She received a master's degree in social history from Georgetown University. Her research interests include long-term care and international perspectives on policies for the aging.

STEPHEN A. GROSSMAN

Mr. Grossman is deputy assistant secretary for health (planning and evaluation) in the U.S. Public Health Service, Department of Health and Human Services (HHS), where he oversees all policy functions and serves as advisor to the assistant secretary for health. Before joining HHS, Grossman was health director and counsel for the Senate Committee on Labor and Human Resources and served as minority counsel to the Senate Subcommittee on Health and Scientific Research.

EDWARD F. HOWARD

Mr. Howard is public policy coordinator at the Villers Foundation. Howard was general counsel at the U.S. House of Representatives Select Committee on Aging under the chairmanship of Rep. Claude Pepper (D-FL) and served as general counsel at the National Council on the Aging. Villers is primarily concerned with issues affecting low-income older Americans, particularly their health care needs. In cooperation with the American Association of Retired Persons, Villers has launched Long Term Care '88, an effort to make long-term care a major issue in the 1988 presidential campaign.

Karen Ignagni

Ms. Ignagni is assistant director of the Department of Occupational Safety, Health, and Social Security at the AFL-CIO, where she is responsible for all health care policy issues. Before joining the American Federation of Labor, she was a professional staff member on the U.S. Senate Labor and Human Resources Committee. Ignagni also served as research director and later as assistant director of the Committee for National Health Insurance and as a health care research analyst in the U.S. Department of Health, Education and Welfare.

Laurence F. Lane

Mr. Lane is vice president for regulatory affairs at InSpeech, Inc., a national rehabilitation services corporation. Lane formerly served as director for special programs at the American Health Care Association, where he chaired a coalition that sponsored three national conferences on private long-term care insurance. Lane has written extensively on the merits of private financing of long-term care. He served as the long-term care technical resource person for the 1981 White House Conference on Aging and managed its mini-conference on long-term care.

F. Peter Libassi

Mr. Libassi served as chairman of the Connecticut Commission on Private and Public Responsibilities for Financing Long-Term Care for the Elderly. He is senior vice president at The Travelers Companies and a member of the Committee on an Aging Society of the National Academy of Science, the Commonwealth Fund Commission for the Elderly Living Alone, and the board of directors for Alliance for Aging Research. He also served on the U.S. Department of Health and Human Services' Task Force on Long Term Health Care Policies.

Stephen R. McConnell

Dr. McConnell is coordinator of Long Term Care '88, a national campaign organized by the American Association of Retired Persons and the Villers Foundation to place long-term care on the presidential campaign agenda. Until recently, he was staff director of the U.S. Senate Special Committee on Aging. From 1980–1984, McConnell was a professional staff member on the U.S. House of Representatives Select Committee on Aging, where he handled policy analysis and legislation pertaining to employment and health.

JOHN J. MCCORMACK

Mr. McCormack is an executive vice president of Teachers Insurance and Annuity Association-College Retirement Equities Fund (TIAA-CREF), where he directs the college services area. This area includes the product research and development division, which is responsible for defining, developing, and monitoring the implementation of new insurance products.

JANET A. MYDER

Ms. Myder is director of special programs at the American Health Care Association (AHCA), where she manages programs on private long-term care insurance development and consumer relations. Before joining AHCA, she was deputy director of the Office of Legislative Liaison and Research at the National Council of Senior Citizens, where she analyzed the impact of federal policy on the health care needs of the aged. Before entering the public policy area, Myder was a physical therapist for 12 years.

THOMAS O'BRIEN

Dr. O'Brien is dean of the School of Management at the University of Massachusetts in Amherst. He serves as chairman of the Commission on Long-Term Care, a study funded by the Carnegie Corporation of New York to establish long-term care insurance for college and university faculty and staff. Until recently, O'Brien was financial vice president for Harvard University. He previously served as director of state planning and management for the Commonwealth of Massachusetts, was a White House Fellow, and served as special assistant to George Romney, then-Secretary of Housing and Urban Development.

JOHN C. ROTHER

Mr. Rother is director of the Legislation, Research, and Public Policy Division of the American Association of Retired Persons (AARP), where he is responsible for federal and state legislative advocacy activities, the Public Policy Institute, and the Voter Education Fund. Before joining AARP in 1984, Rother served as staff director and chief counsel for the U.S. Senate Special Committee on Aging. He also served as special counsel for labor and health issues to former Sen. Jacob Javits (R-NY). Prior to his Capitol Hill experience, Rother was an appellate litigator for the National Labor Relations Board and worked in the U.S. Department of Health and Human Services' Office for Civil Rights.

THERESA VARNER

Ms. Varner is a health policy analyst in the Public Policy Institute at the American Association of Retired Persons. She received a master's degree in social work and a master's degree in English literature from the University of Alabama. Her research interests include Medicare beneficiary liability and catastrophic health care coverage.

BRUCE C. VLADECK

Dr. Vladeck is president of the United Hospital Fund of New York. He previously served as assistant vice president of the Robert Wood Johnson Foundation and as assistant commissioner for health planning and resources development of the New Jersey State Department of Health. He is a member of the Prospective Payment Assessment Commission, the Board of Directors of the New York City Health and Hospitals Corporation, the New York State Council of Health Care Financing, and the Institute of Medicine, National Academy of Sciences.

RICHARD WOODBURY

Mr. Woodbury is a doctoral candidate in economics at Harvard University. He graduated from Williams College in Williamstown, Massachusetts.

LEON WYSZEWIANSKI

Dr. Wyszewianski is an associate professor in the Department of Health Services Management and Policy at the University of Michigan's School of Public Health. His research and publications cover a broad spectrum of health care delivery and health policy topics, much of which focuses on high-cost illnesses and catastrophic health care expenditures.

PART ONE
WHY ARE CATASTROPHIC AND LONG-TERM HEALTH CARE PUBLIC POLICY ISSUES?

Major social and demographic trends in America are leading federal lawmakers and other policymakers to a new focus in the health care field: what should be the public and/or private response to the plight of millions of Americans who face possible financial ruin from catastrophic health care expenses?

The trends that have sparked the debate over catastrophic health care expenses include the aging of the population and the increasing number of both working and nonworking Americans without health care insurance or with inadequate coverage.

For the elderly, the catastrophic event can be the need for long-term chronic care in a nursing home—the cost of which threatens the loss of assets and savings even for those who believe they are well-protected by their resources. The urgency of the issue stems from projections that as many as one in every two persons now in their 50s will spend some time in a nursing home in their remaining lifetime.

For the nonelderly, civilian, nonagricultural, uninsured population—whose numbers grew from 30.3 million in 1982 to nearly 35 million in 1986—even relatively modest expenditures on health care can be catastrophic.

To address one part of this problem—catastrophic expenses of the elderly for acute health care needs, such as lengthy stays in a hospital, the 100th Congress has broadened Medicare coverage through a new catastrophic insurance program. The program does not, however, address the long-term care issue, although other congressional proposals have been introduced to deal with the problem. Lawmakers have also proposed legislation requiring employers to provide at least a minimum health benefit package for most workers and their dependents. Part One of *Where Coverage Ends: Catastrophic Illness and Long-Term Health Care Costs* provides an overview of the financing issues relating to catastrophic health care expenses for the elderly and nonelderly populations.

In chapter I, Stephen McConnell focuses principally on long-term care: public opinion on the issue, business community involvement,

1

congressional actions, and political ramifications in the 1988 presidential race. McConnell points out that long-term care has not been on the public agenda until recently because it has long been considered an obligation of families, with adult daughters being the primary caregivers. With more women working, McConnell says, trying to care for infirm elders in the home has become more difficult.

McConnell argues that the debate over the catastrophic health insurance legislation has also drawn more public attention to the lack of coverage for long-term care in that program and under Medicare in general. Reporting on polls taken of the public and of businesses, he finds that there is heightened interest in the issue. Most Americans want a government program to address the problem, he contends, and an increasing number of businesses are considering offering long-term care as an employee benefit.

After reviewing various congressional proposals that would establish public programs or that would provide incentives to the private sector to market long-term care insurance, McConnell notes that actual action in Congress has been slow because of fears about the cost. Congress is waiting, he says, to see where public opinion is going and what will happen in the private insurance area.

McConnell concludes with a look at the positions of the 1988 presidential candidates on long-term care. The politicians are also wary about cost, he says, and are uncertain of political support. McConnell predicts, however, that long-term care will continue to be a major issue during the next few years.

In chapter II the discussion among the forum participants focuses on the part that families play in providing long-term care for their relatives and on their need for support in meeting this obligation. Representatives of firms that have taken the initiative in providing group long-term coverage explain how their insurance policies are being financed, discuss how employees are responding to the policies, and offer suggestions on ways to educate workers about this important issue.

I. The Emerging Politics of Catastrophic and Long-Term Care Policy

REMARKS OF STEPHEN R. MCCONNELL

Introduction

To begin, I will give an overview of long-term care and why it is a public policy issue. Then I will review how the public views the issue; how Congress and the business community are dealing with the issue; and, finally, how the issue is being approached by the 1988 presidential candidates. I will focus principally on long-term care, although I will discuss some aspects of broader catastrophic coverage.

In June 1988 Congress passed legislation to aid the elderly in financing catastrophic health care expenses.* Essentially, this legislation offers protection against acute-care catastrophic costs, with a cap on out-of-pocket expenses. Thus, if you spend greater than the cap amount, you are protected through this new benefit, financed through an increase in the Medicare Part B premium.**

While this legislation offers important coverage for the elderly, 8 out of 10 dollars spent by the elderly for catastrophic care will not be covered by this legislation. The reason: the vast bulk of catastrophic costs for the elderly is for long-term, chronic care.

It is important to keep in mind that one in two people in their 50s will, during their remaining lifetime, spend some time in a nursing home; one in four will spend a year or more in a nursing home. If they are there for chronic care, none of the costs would be covered by this catastrophic insurance program or by basic Medicare benefits.

Before going on, I should mention something about my background. I generally wear three hats: one, I am an advocate of long-term care, having spent most of my career in the field of aging, and I am now working on a campaign to try to get long-term care onto the national agenda. Second, I am something of an analyst on this issue. And, third, I am a family member who deals with the problem of long-term care. My father has had a major stroke and is a long-term care patient.

---

*Editor's note: For a complete description of the Medicare Catastrophic Coverage Act, as enacted by Congress in June 1988, see Appendix C.

**Editor's note: Medicare Part B, also called Medicare Supplementary Medical Insurance (SMI), provides insurance coverage for physician services and outpatient medical care as well as some hospital services not paid by the Part A Hospital Insurance Program.

What is long-term care? In my father's case, he is severely disabled and living at home. My mother is caring for him and is providing day-to-day care—helping him get dressed, feeding him, and providing him with a variety of nonmedical services.

Long-term care for Betty Stevens is nursing home care for both of her parents, who are ages 84 and 79. It is costing $5,000 a month, and she had to sell her parents' home and deplete her savings in order to help pay for that care. For Mrs. Brannigan, who is 94, long-term care is provided by her son, Ray Brannigan, 72.

I mention these examples because sometimes we talk about statistics and it is hard to get a sense of what it is we are really talking about. Long-term care is chronic care requiring some medical but mostly social services that can be provided in institutions or at home, and it includes everything from meal preparation to more detailed kinds of social services.

There are about 8 million elderly persons in the United States who have some degree of chronic dependency requiring long-term care, and about 1.5 million who are in nursing homes. Long-term care has traditionally been provided informally, mostly by the adult children of aged parents.

When I was in China a few years ago, I was struck by the fact that there were very few nursing homes: in cities with populations of 11 or 12 million there were only one or two nursing homes, and those were principally for men who never married, who did not have families. For the most part, Chinese families provide long-term care services for the aged.

The same is true in this country. More than two-thirds of the long-term care provided for the elderly is provided by families. Generally, the care is provided by the eldest daughter or daughter-in-law. In my family, my father is cared for mostly by my mother. We built a little apartment on my sister's house and my parents live there. My sister's family helps provide some of the care.

Long-Term Care as a Public Policy Issue

Although catastrophic and long-term care have historically been handled privately, both are rapidly becoming public problems. My evidence for this assertion comes, in part, from my seven years working with Congress, for both the House and Senate Aging Committees. During that time, there was a surprising dearth of mail on the issues of catastrophic or long-term care. The reason is that, generally, long-term care has been considered to be a family obligation. Families

4

provided this care out of a sense of responsibility and, in some cases, out of guilt. Most feel that "my parents cared for me; I should, in turn, care for them." Another reason that this issue has not been on the public agenda is that it is a nonmedical problem. As a result, there are no groups of powerful service providers who lobby for benefits in this area. Additionally, in the past, flexibility in Medicare and Medicaid rules has made it possible to absorb some of the cost of long-term care by permitting prolonged hospital stays.

While the problem has been viewed as a private concern in the past, the situation is changing dramatically. First, many members of Congress and increasing numbers of the public have started to recognize that long-term care is not covered by the new catastrophic health care legislation.

If the catastrophic insurance legislation has done anything, it has alerted people to what is not protected. Virtually every news article that has been written about the legislation has included a piece about the lack of coverage for long-term care.

Second, attention is shifting to long-term care because of the growth of the elderly population. The oldest part of the population—the old-old, age 85 and older—are now the fastest-growing segment of the population, increasing at twice the rate of younger age groups.

Third, improved technology has also brought this issue to the surface. We now can keep people alive longer, which means that the need for long-term care is more evident.

Fourth, there have been changes in work patterns. As more and more women enter the labor force, they are less available to care for aged parents. Because adult daughters provide the bulk of long-term care services, their need to work creates strains and stresses on the family. These stresses are beginning to be expressed publicly.

And, finally, a growing group of health care providers—long-term care providers—are now exercising their muscles both on Capitol Hill and through public opinion, to get some protection for long-term care. The National Association for Home Care, the American Association of Homes for the Aging, and the American Health Care Association are just three organizations that have grown rapidly in the last few years, and are helping to bring greater public attention to this issue.

Public Opinion

As a result of these forces, public opinion is changing. I would like to report on a nationwide poll conducted for the American Association

5

of Retired Persons (AARP) and the Villers Foundation during the summer of 1987. The poll of 1,000 voting-age Americans focused on long-term care, how people are viewing this problem, and what they want done about it.

The poll results are rather striking. First, 60 percent of Americans have had some experience with long-term care. One-half of these have had experience in their own families, and another 15 percent or so have had experience through a very close friend. Another 20 percent expect to face the problem within the next five years.

Thus, 80 percent of the population either has had some experience with long-term care or expects to in the next five years. These numbers are staggering. Even among the youngest group surveyed, the 18- to 29-age group, one-third had had some direct experience with long-term care.

The second finding in this poll is that long-term care is a major financial and emotional concern. Americans are confronting both the emotional and economic problems associated with long-term care. Three-fourths of the people in this poll said it would be "a major sacrifice or impossible" to pay one year of the cost of nursing home care. Two-thirds said that they would feel guilty about putting an aged parent in a nursing home. Most people polled are afraid of becoming a burden to their children, but they realize that major conflicts arise around the problem of long-term care.

The third finding is that six out of seven Americans want a government program to address this problem. Most are aware that Medicare does not cover long-term care and want the government to address the issue in some way. This response came from both Democrats and Republicans. Eighty-two percent of Republicans said that they felt it was time for the government to step in on this issue.

And, finally, according to the poll, Americans are willing to pay additional taxes for a government program. By a 5-to-2 margin, they were willing to pay amounts that varied according to their income, but amounts that were calculated to reflect at least a moderate amount of the cost that would be incurred by a government long-term care program.

The real test of the public saliency of an issue for many of us comes from our personal experiences. For me, the real test was when I was in California at my parents' 50th wedding anniversary. During a program that reviewed my parents' lives, there was a brief description of what each of their four children is doing. When it was mentioned that I am working to help put the issue of long-term care on the presidential agenda, spontaneous applause broke out. That may be more convincing than any national poll—and much more gratifying.

I should add that other polls conducted in the last two years show that people are interested in seeing something done about long-term care, particularly for the elderly. These polls indicate that most people want the government to step in and that there is some willingness to pay additional taxes for it. In sum, the problem of long-term care is very rapidly emerging as a public policy problem.

Employers Begin to Focus on Long-Term Care

The business community is awakening to the problems of catastrophic and long-term care, but there is reluctance to move very far, or very fast.

In a recent survey of their own employees, The Travelers Insurance Companies found that a large number are acting as long-term caregivers. Studies by IBM and other companies have found very similar results.

The aging of the work force and the growing number of retirees are causing the business community to begin to pay attention to long-term care. IBM recently announced the "Elder Care Program," a nationwide referral and assessment program for long-term care, established in early 1988. The IBM program is not a benefit, but is a recognition that long-term care is a problem confronting more and more employees and retirees.

I would like to report briefly on some results of a survey of 145 Fortune 1000 companies, done over a two-month period in the summer of 1987 by the Washington Business Group on Health. It was funded by The Travelers and Alcoa Foundations, American Express, and J.C. Penney.*

The results are comparable to those of a confidential survey done for the insurance industry, which provides some additional validation of the results. First, the survey found that interest in long-term care benefits is high, but action today among employers is only modest. More than a third of the companies surveyed have had or are having internal discussions and have talked to insurers about long-term care. An additional one-fifth of the companies plan to have discussions about this issue in the next few years. Only seven companies have

---

*Editor's note: The report, *Corporate Perspective on Long-Term Care—Survey Report*, was published December 1987 by the Washington Business Group on Health.

conducted surveys of their employees similar to those Travelers and IBM, and six have discussed this problem with their unions.

The motivation for companies to look into this issue appears to be coming mostly from the increased publicity about long-term care and from staff within the companies' benefits departments. There was some mention that employees and unions are placing some demands on employers to take action on long-term care, but that is not the major reason that employers are beginning to look at the issue.

One-half of the employers surveyed recognized that chronic care is being paid for through acute-care benefits. The preferred benefit arrangement for long-term care among the employers surveyed was "employee-pay-all." Two-thirds of the employers said that they were interested, strongly or somewhat, in employee-pay-all benefits. Only six were interested in employer-pay-all benefits. Most would offer a benefit only through insurance companies rather than through self-insurance, which might be because companies are afraid of the liability, as are some insurance companies.

The likelihood of offering long-term care benefits, according to the survey, was relatively high. For employee-pay-all benefits, one-half of the employers said that it was "probable" that they would offer a benefit in the next five years; 22 (15 percent) of the 145 companies said that it was "highly probable" they would offer some base of benefits.

The barriers to offering long-term care protection mentioned were the high price and administrative costs, the unavailability of products, and the lack of employee interest.

The conclusion from this survey is that business, like the public, is beginning to recognize that long-term care is an issue. Employers are starting to look into it, but very little has been put into place at the present time. In fact, only about 10 percent of the companies said that their preretirement planning programs included information on long-term care.

Congressional Action Unclear

Now that Congress has dealt with the catastrophic insurance legislation for the elderly, it will be confronted with long-term care issues. While Congress is acknowledging these issues, there is still a question as to what is likely to happen in the future.

There is growing pressure to address the issue of access to health care for the uninsured, which is the focus of the mandated benefits legislation sponsored by Sen. Edward M. Kennedy (D-MA).* With 37 million people uninsured, and with that number growing by roughly one million each year, there is going to be increasing pressure on Congress to act. Some people have commented that Sen. Kennedy has found the three employers who like this idea, and those three have testified, so there may not be any more hearings until they can find more employers in support of this legislation. Nonetheless, there is increasing public pressure to address the broad issue of catastrophic coverage for the uninsured.

In the long-term care area, the focus in Congress has principally been on the issue of quality, the public outcry has been over quality problems in nursing homes. Again, if the poll results are accurate, and if the growing pressures on families to deal with long-term care continue, Congress will have to address more than the quality issue. There is some movement in Congress now.

The legislation sponsored by Rep. Claude Pepper (D-FL) to extend Medicare to provide chronic-care benefits at home for children, the elderly, and the disabled was defeated in June 1988.

Sen. Dave Durenberger (R-MN) and Rep. Ron Wyden (D-OR) each has introduced legislation that would contribute to the attractiveness of private insurance (S. 1739 and H.R. 3438, respectively). Sen. Durenberger's bill would allow favorable tax treatment of the so-called "inside buildup" of long-term care insurance reserves. Rep. Wyden's bill would provide favorable tax treatment for premiums paid by employers for long-term care insurance. The merits of such approaches are being debated by a growing number of members of Congress.

Sen. John Chafee (R-RI) has introduced a home care bill (S. 1673) that would modify Medicaid and open it up to home care benefits. Rep. Edward Roybal (D-CA) has introduced a comprehensive health bill that would provide long-term care benefits through Medicare (H.R. 200).

Other developments include the following.

- The Medicare Catastrophic Coverage Act of 1988 provides for a bipartisan commission to report back to Congress within six months on long-term care coverage for people of all ages, with an emphasis on the social insurance approach. Six months after that, the commission must propose

---

*Editor's note: The Minimum Health Benefits for All Workers Act (S. 1265) would require employers to provide at least a minimum health benefit package for most workers and their dependents.

9

solutions to health care problems in general, not just long-term care. So there will be some additional attention to this issue as a result of yet another congressional task force.

- Reporting its findings in September 1987, the Department of Health and Human Services (HHS) Task Force on Long-Term Health Care Policies encouraged the use of the tax code for both state and federal long-term care benefits.*

- There may be an issue on the ballot in California to provide subsidies for low-income people who buy long-term care insurance.

Notwithstanding the above, it is important to note that none of the major tax-writing committees in Congress which have jurisdiction over the long-term care issue has made any significant commitment to addressing it. The reason: there is a good deal of fear about the cost of long-term care. More and more individual members of Congress, however, are putting legislation together.

Sen. George Mitchell (D-ME), chairman of the Senate Finance Subcommittee on Health, has introduced The Long-Term Care Assistance Act of 1988 (S.2306).** Sen. John Heinz (R-PA), also a member of the Senate Finance Committee, is preparing legislation. I mentioned Sen. Chafee's bill, and I suspect Sen. Bill Bradley (D-NJ) will be involved in developing some long-term care legislation.

In sum, Congress is waiting to determine what public opinion will be and what will happen in the private insurance area. At the same time, there is growing public pressure, which is likely to increase as more people realize what the catastrophic insurance legislation does and does *not* cover.

Presidential Election Politics and Long-Term Care

All of the 1988 presidential candidates have made a commitment to address long-term care in some form. Governor Michael Dukakis supports the catastrophic health care legislation, although he cautions against requiring Medicare beneficiaries to pay an ever-increasing share of program costs. He also favored the long-term care bill (H.R. 3436) introduced by Rep. Claude Pepper (D-FL), which would

---

*Editor's note: See U.S. Department of Health and Human Services, *Report to Congress and the Secretary by the Task Force on Long-Term Health Care Policies*, executive summary, Appendix B.

**Editor's note: This bill is considered unique in that it establishes a partnership between the private sector and government by providing stop-loss coverage through the expansion of public programs and encouraging a private insurance market.

have expanded the Medicare program to cover home care services. Reverend Jesse Jackson has endorsed a national health care program that would build on the current Medicare program but would be universal and comprehensive. Vice President George Bush has proposed a program to provide tax incentives for the purchase of long-term care insurance and allow for conversion of IRAs, savings accounts, and life insurance to finance long-term care.

In the national poll that I discussed earlier, a majority of Americans said that they would be more likely to vote for a candidate who supports a long-term care program and, conversely, would vote against a candidate who opposed long-term care coverage. The poll also makes it clear that there is a very positive image that goes with support for a long-term care program. By a three-to-one margin, respondents reject the notion that a candidate would be considered a "big spender" if he supported a long-term care program. By the same margin, they agreed that candidates supporting long-term care show "leadership vision."

The sentiment that prevails as you look at the poll results is that this is a *family issue*. With the large numbers of people who have had experience with long-term care, development of a long-term care program is not something we are doing to help somebody else out there. The feeling is: "It would help me and my family." To the extent that this family message is communicated to the candidates, it is going to be compelling.

The problems for candidates on the long-term care issue and the reason that they are somewhat wary is, first, the cost. Some of this is the fear of a new government program, but it is mostly a fear of raising taxes, especially given the drop in the financial market in the fall of 1987.

The second reason for the hesitancy is the uncertainty of political support. The poll results are clear, but they have to be reinforced by people insisting that this is an issue that must take precedence over many others the candidates have to address.

Health issues historically have not been particularly exciting material for political campaigns, and that causes candidates to be cautious.

And, finally, there is concern about the intergenerational aspect. Candidates may hesitate to talk about providing long-term care for the elderly and taxing the young to pay for it.

The plus for candidates is that this is a family issue that affects most Americans. It carries a positive image. At least until the stock market crash, no major issues had surfaced in this election. With that void, an issue like long-term care, to the extent it gets substantial public support, could emerge more frequently on the agenda.

The question, then, is how far up on the presidential agendas will this issue rise?

Conclusion

Long-term care is emerging as an item for the national agenda because of demographic and work force changes, because of catastrophic insurance legislation which has heightened public awareness, and because there is a sense of pressure from families that there is a need for some assistance on this problem.

Employers and insurers are dangling their toes in the water. The Congress is looking at the issue and the presidential candidates are looking at it.

The economy could dampen any movement toward a major government approach to long-term care, but I doubt that there is anything that will dampen the rising concern about the problem among families.

II. Part One Discussion

A Family or Societal Responsibility?

MR. JACKSON: There was continual reference throughout your comments to the burdens on the family. This is true in The Travelers' survey, for example. Also you refer to China, where the families handle much of this. My concern is about the one-third of the younger generation that did not feel guilty about putting their parents in a nursing home.

I wonder about the psychological impact on our entire culture and the way we live if we try to pawn off a family responsibility onto society. I have noticed, for example, the contrast between the last five or ten years and the 1930s, when everybody helped other people even though nobody had very much. Today you can walk down K Street in Washington and pass people who are hungry and you just walk by, and the reason is that the government takes care of them.

It is one thing to take the burden of caring for the poor off of the individual, although I think you rob people of the joy of contributing to someone else's welfare, when you just tax. After all, you don't get much psychological pleasure out of paying a tax even if you know that half of it is going to poor people. What happens when you remove this family obligation?

MR. McCONNELL: I don't think anybody who is dealing with this issue would remove the family obligation. Even if we tried, we could not really do that, but it would also be very bad policy to try. What is driving the concern about this issue is the recognition that families are being increasingly burdened, not just by caring for their parents, but by the fact that more and more women who are middle-aged and have to work for a variety of reasons, are caught in this bind between their job and caring for their aged parents. Also driving this issue is the fact that some people have to spend-down into poverty and lose everything that they have saved throughout their lives to cover long-term care, while another family who was lucky can pass a large inheritance to the next generation.

Long-term care is not just a matter of providing nursing home care where it is appropriate; it also involves providing assistance at home so that people can continue to work and so the family caregivers do not break down. Any program must support family care, not replace it.

13

The problem is often referred to as the "woodwork effect"—that if you offer a benefit, people will come out of the woodwork, and the public program will replace what had been provided privately.

A comparison was done between Massachusetts, which is very benefit-rich, and a southern state that has limited benefits. It was found that elderly people got more care in Massachusetts, but that the families were as involved and provided as much care as they did in the southern state. This suggests that providing coverage can improve the care, but the family does not simply back away from their responsibility.

Employer Initiatives in Group Long-Term Care Policies

Ms. GAGLIARDI: American Express introduced a group long-term care policy covering our employees, beginning January 1, 1988. Their parents and in-laws will be eligible for the program, and then probably later in the first quarter of 1988, we will offer it to retirees.

We have conducted extensive employee focus groups this year in order to determine interest in this subject. Contrary to one of the results in the survey that you mentioned, we found that there was enormously high employee interest, even among the relatively young employee population, because they do feel it is their problem. Many of those employees were already providing care for elderly relatives, and so they saw it as a great step forward. The benefit includes care in a nursing home and also home health care.

QUESTION FROM THE AUDIENCE: How would it be financed?

Ms. GAGLIARDI: It is going to be insured through Travelers.

QUESTION FROM THE AUDIENCE: Employer paid or employee paid?

Ms. GAGLIARDI: It is going to be paid for by the employee, at least initially. And the rates are very, very reasonable if you manage to sign up when you are young.

MR. McCONNELL: That will be the test.

Ms. GAGLIARDI: It sure will be. But based on the interest that we find, we expect the younger employees to enroll because they see this not only for themselves down the road, but also for the remote possibility that they might need it sooner.

Ms. YOUNG: What do you mean by young? Is young 20, or is young 40?

14

Ms. GAGLIARDI: 30. Between 30 and 40.

MR. McCONNELL: Looking at our poll results, interest seems to increase at 30.

MR. O'BRIEN: Steve, you did not talk separately about home care. Were you talking about both home and nursing home care?

MR. McCONNELL: Long-term care really includes both nursing home care and home care. The poll shows that most people would want coverage for home care as well as nursing home care. The big costs, of course, are generally in the nursing home care area, but the big need—the biggest needs—are for care at home.

Ms. SCHAEFFER: You can add John Hancock to your list of employers who are offering long-term care insurance to their employees. An enormous amount of interest was expressed at our benefit fair last year. Many were on the young side, as you have suggested. So, we are quite anxious to find out how many apply.

The insurance is employer-pay-all as part of our flexible benefits plan, and we are using ADL criteria to determine eligibility for benefits in a nursing home or in the person's own home. As you point out, the cost of the benefits is a lot greater in the nursing home, but the frequency of utilization is much greater in the home. So, we are anticipating a greater portion of our claim costs to be attributable to the home.

Ms. YOUNG: Have any of the researchers looked at the demographics? The world has changed a lot since the 1930s. What will happen, for instance, if 50 percent of the population is divorced. Are you going to wind up with one or both elderly parents having had very little contact with their children? I see a scenario in which there are a large number of elderly gentlemen who are not going to be taken care of by daughters-in-law whom they have never met before becoming dependent. These women are not going to quit their jobs to take care of these gentlemen.

Everybody is talking about whether or not we are going to have people throwing their burdens onto public programs if such programs are developed, but the question right now is whether people consider it to be their burden.

Attitudes of the Younger Generation

MR. McCONNELL: There are two parts to your question. One is, what is happening to the attitudes among the younger generation,

15

vis-à-vis the old. The two people who spoke about their benefit plans suggested that those young people are very interested in this for their parents and for themselves.

MS. YOUNG: But those are people who are now 35 and 40.

MR. MCCONNELL: That's true. In the research that I'm aware of, the commitment to caring for the aged, so-called filial responsibility, has not changed substantially over time. There is this notion that in the old days we took care of our parents, and today we dump them off. The statistics just do not support that. Increasingly, however, there is less time for caregiving. For example, women who are working have less time to care for aged parents. But there is still a lot of intergenerational transfer of contact and money.

The second part of your question pertains to changing demographics. With more women in the work force, fewer children per family, a rise in childless families, and a high divorce rate, there simply will be an increased demand for a public response to this issue.

I do not think that attitudes concerning support for parents are changing dramatically. It is incumbent on any public policy development to ensure that we do not encourage families to abandon their aged parents.

MR. MCCORMACK: Did you mention that in countries like China as many as one-third of the men were single?

MR. MCCONNELL: I made the observation that even in Chinese cities with very, very large populations, there were only a handful of nursing homes—perhaps one or two—and those were typically for men who never married. I raised that point not as a way of saying that that is what we used to be like, but to show that more traditional societies, where the family provides the care, are not all that different from this country.

Raising the Awareness of Employees

MR. MCCORMACK: It has been said that American Express and John Hancock will be offering long-term care coverage to their employees. American Express mentioned a focus group. In bringing the issue to the attention of your employees, how much of an educational role did you play?

Did you pique the interest of the 30-year-olds by raising the issue, or were they coming to you saying "We really ought to, as an organization, be doing something for our employees, about this di-

16

lemma?" How much of a role did you, as employers, play in creating interest in the issue?

Ms. GAGLIARDI: At American Express we felt that there was a degree of education that we had to go through to enable employees to react intelligently to some of the questions we were posing. It was not so much a matter of sparking their interest as of bringing them the kinds of statistics that we have all heard today. We found that enough employees had had the caregiver experience within their own family that they were sufficiently aware of the need for this kind of program.

Ms. SCHAEFFER: At John Hancock, we had some focus groups and we also participated in a private insurance survey earlier this year, but we did not survey our own employees. We considered them as part of the same population surveyed in the studies mentioned.

The way we are handling it in the introduction phase is through a very careful education campaign. We are very careful not to sell or press people to sign up. Rather it is an education in awareness.

MR. CRABTREE: I am with the Principal Financial Group, which has its headquarters in Des Moines, Iowa. Our community affairs have to do with the activities and concerns of rural areas.

In these areas health care is a real economic development issue— and a very major concern. As communities shrink, if health care is not available, the community shrinks faster because the elderly leave. When they leave, they take dollars with them. Particularly in rural Iowa and in the surrounding states, the people who leave are those who have the most money.

There has been a growing awareness that not only is this a health care issue, it is a long-term care issue. The development commission and the community development organizations are all trying to figure out how they can have a role. In a sense, this speaks to the previous question about whether there have been surveys to find out if families are available to provide care. The fact is, everybody knows they are not.

The kids left a long time ago, and the people who remain do not have family available. If there is no institution to which they can relate, they leave.

A growing number of people are concerned about helping these people stay in their towns. While this concern no doubt springs from a genuine desire to help, it also reflects a sense that these communities are going to dry up faster if health and long-term care facilities are not available.

If we can figure out how to help people in rural areas, they can become very important assets for getting things done.

Ms. MYDER: The fact that the participation of women in the work force has shifted some of the burden for long-term care either outside of the family or outside of the home is very significant. It certainly is one of the main reasons that we are so concerned about financing long-term care. However, I caution those who are tempted to increase the family's role in caregiving not to assume that the burden was any easier to bear when women were in the home taking care of elderly family members. It was probably just as great. We now may be more aware of the burdens, but let us not assume that it was any easier then than it is now.

PART TWO
A SEARCH FOR DEFINITIONS AND SOLUTIONS

In Part Two we turn to an examination of what constitutes "catastrophic" health expenditures both for the population as a whole and for the elderly. Leon Wyszewianski makes a case in chapter III for formulating a definition of catastrophic health expenditures that is "based on clear conceptual distinctions" and attempts to reflect social values and goals. Chapter IV, an EBRI analysis by Deborah Chollet and Charles Betley, discusses the issue in terms of the non-elderly population.

Professor Wyszewianski distinguishes between "financially catastrophic cases," situations in which health care expenses exceed a family's ability to pay, and "high-cost cases," in which total health care expenditures exceed a certain amount. Wyszewianski argues that most existing catastrophic insurance programs tend to equate high-cost cases with financially catastrophic ones and to rely on a "stop-loss approach," in which protection against catastrophic expenses becomes available only after basic coverage is exhausted. This type of approach, he adds, considers a health expenditure as truly catastrophic only if it is a large expense.

Wyszewianski maintains, however, that expense in relation to ability to pay must be considered if people are to be protected against severe financial consequences. Wyszewianski finds that where disposable income is so limited that even a relatively small health care cost exceeds the ability to pay, the need for protection is more pressing than it is for the traditional targets of catastrophic programs.

If a catastrophic expenditure is defined as one that exceeds ability to pay, Wyszewianski says, the questions that must be asked are: what is "ability to pay" and what are "health care expenditures?"

How income and assets are measured for the purpose of defining ability to pay tells us how much we as a society are prepared to let a person's or family's standard of living decline before relief is provided, Wyszewianski argues. He asks whether we believe that people must exhaust their income and assets and become destitute before they can become eligible for catastrophic care protection.

Wyszewianski makes a case for including expenditures for long-term care in the definition of health care expenditures, because to exclude such expenses runs counter, he says, to the basic goals of catastrophic programs to cover expenses that exceed the ability to pay.

In chapter IV Deborah Chollet and Charles Betley point out that although three-quarters of the nonelderly population have private health insurance coverage, not all are fully covered for all types of health care expenses. For uninsured people, any major illness can result in a catastrophic level of health care expense.

Chollet and Betley examine alternative definitions of catastrophic health care costs and the implications of those definitions for calculating the number of people believed to be at risk of incurring catastrophic expenses. They echo Wyszewianski's point that defining catastrophic costs by reference to an absolute dollar limit fails to account for differences among families in ability to finance health care. Although the problem could be resolved by using a percentage-of-family-income definition instead, this formula could be administratively difficult for private or public health insurers. By any definition, Chollet and Betley conclude, families in poverty are more likely to have catastrophic levels of uninsured health care expenses than are nonpoor families.

In chapter V, John Rother, Mary Jo Gibson, and Theresa Varner attempt to develop a framework for a comprehensive long-term care social insurance program.

They argue that the term "catastrophic" used in connection with the Medicare Catastrophic Coverage Act of 1988 a misnomer since the program does not cover long-term care. Nursing home stays, they say, account for over 80 percent of the expense incurred by older persons, who must spend more than $2,000 out-of-pocket per year.

The authors describe a proposal for a long-term care social insurance program that was developed in 1987 by the American Association of Retired Persons (AARP), the Villers Foundation, and the Older Women's League. The proposed program, built on an expansion of Medicare, would provide community-based and institutional care services to persons who are severely disabled. Separate financing mechanisms would be developed for future retirees and for those currently retired.*

In chapter VI forum participants discuss long-term care as posing a risk not only for the individual but for the family, and for middle-

---

*Public and private roles in financing catastrophic and long-term care are the subject of Part IV.

20

aged and younger people as well as the elderly. They debate issues involved in building an infrastructure and developing financing mechanisms.

III. Catastrophic Health Expenditures: Toward a Working Definition

PAPER BY LEON WYSZEWIANSKI

Introduction

The provision of coverage for catastrophic health care expenditures is once again a visible public policy issue. Yet, despite the intense current interest in the issue and the many proposals for catastrophic health care coverage that have been made periodically for more than three decades—including those that resulted in several states enacting their own catastrophic health insurance programs (Van Ellet, 1981)—fundamental issues of definition remain unresolved.

What follows makes a case for formulating a definition of catastrophic health expenditures that is based on clear conceptual distinctions, takes into account some of the empirical findings that bear on those distinctions, and explicitly attempts to reflect pertinent social values and goals.

Defining Catastrophic Health Expenditures

Financially Catastrophic Cases versus High-Cost Cases—There is no widely accepted definition of what a catastrophic health care expenditure is. It is useful to make an explicit distinction between financially catastrophic cases and high-cost ones, where the term *financially catastrophic case* refers specifically to situations in which health care expenditures exceed a person's or a family's ability to pay (Wyszewianski, 1986). "Ability to pay" is specified in relation to third-party coverage and income (or in relation to these two factors plus assets). For example, a health care expenditure might be considered financially catastrophic if out-of-pocket expenditures for health services exceed 15 percent (or 20 or 25 percent) of family income.

The term *high-cost case*, on the other hand, refers to cases for which total health care expenditures exceed a certain amount, such as $10,000 in one year, regardless of the source of payment or the affected person's ability to pay for the care. Although it is often assumed that all high-cost cases are also financially catastrophic, the two categories are not identical. Rather, they are partly overlapping (chart III.1).

23

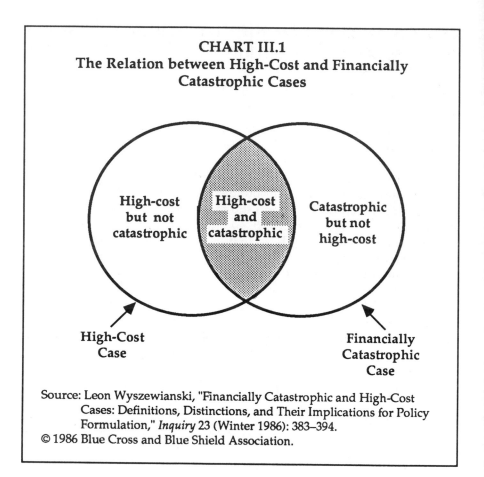

CHART III.1
The Relation between High-Cost and Financially Catastrophic Cases

High-cost but not catastrophic

High-cost and catastrophic

Catastrophic but not high-cost

High-Cost Case

Financially Catastrophic Case

Source: Leon Wyszewianski, "Financially Catastrophic and High-Cost
Cases: Definitions, Distinctions, and Their Implications for Policy
Formulation," *Inquiry* 23 (Winter 1986): 383–394.
© 1986 Blue Cross and Blue Shield Association.

Some financially catastrophic cases are high-cost, but not all are. Similarly, not all high-cost cases are also catastrophic. The degree of overlap between the two categories depends on the individual's ability to pay. For a person who has very comprehensive health insurance coverage with no cost-sharing features, there is virtually no expenditure, no matter how high-cost, that will be catastrophic. At the other extreme, even small health care expenditures can be financially catastrophic for a person with no third-party coverage, a low income, and no assets.

In the context of protecting people against suffering severe financial consequences resulting from expenditures for health care services, it is consistent with most people's understanding of a financially catastrophic expenditure to define it in relation to ability to pay. The meaning and implications of doing so can be illustrated by examining the characteristics of families with financially catastrophic expenditures.

Empirical Findings and Their Implications—The most recent description of the characteristics of families with catastrophic health care expenditures is based on data for a nationally representative group of families from the 1977 National Medical Care Expenditure Survey (Wyszewianski, 1986). The analysis describes three overlapping groups of families: those that spent more than 5, 10, and 20 percent of their income on out-of-pocket health care expenditures. Only expenditures for care received in hospitals or in the offices of physicians and other practitioners were included in the analysis. It therefore specifically excludes expenditures for nursing homes. The findings, summarized briefly in the following paragraphs, are consistent with an earlier report on the characteristics of families that in 1970 had out-of-pocket health care expenditures exceeding 15 percent of their income (Kasper et al., 1975).

Most families with out-of-pocket expenditures for health care representing a relatively large percentage of their income were found to have actually spent small amounts. Even among the families that spent more than 20 percent of their income on health care, over one-fourth had annual out-of-pocket expenditures in 1977 of less than $500, and nearly half spent less than $1,000. Only 9 percent had annual out-of-pocket expenditures above $4,000.

Relatively small amounts account for a substantial proportion of many of these families' incomes because those incomes are comparatively low: among families spending more than 20 percent of their income on out-of-pocket health care expenditures, only 6 percent had incomes above $12,000 (in 1977 dollars) and 66 percent were below the poverty level. By contrast, 54 percent of *all* families had incomes over $12,000 and only 15 percent were below the poverty level.

In addition to their low incomes, families with catastrophic expenditures had inadequate third-party coverage. On average, those with out-of-pocket expenditures representing 20 percent of their income paid directly for 41 percent of their total health care bill, significantly above the average 31 percent paid by all families. In addition, families with high out-of-pocket expenditures in relation to their income had a significantly smaller percentage of their total expenditures covered by Medicaid, suggesting that these families by and large do not qualify for Medicaid coverage, even though two-thirds were below the poverty line. These families were also found to be more

25

likely to be headed by an unemployed person, and a disproportionate number were headed by someone 65 or older.

Overall, the analysis suggests that most families whose out-of-pocket health services expenditures are high in relation to their incomes find themselves in that predicament not so much because of high-cost illnesses but more fundamentally because of their low incomes and a lack of basic health care coverage. Yet, to date, catastrophic coverage programs and proposals have not addressed the specific needs suggested by these findings.

Characteristics of Past Definitions

The Stop-Loss Approach—Rather than seeing catastrophic health care coverage as a means to protect individuals and families from incurring health services expenditures that greatly exceed their ability to pay, many catastrophic coverage programs and proposals are based on the more narrow and not always explicitly stated goal of offering protection to victims of devastating diseases or injuries. Such programs are intended for situations that require care that is so costly that either coverage limits are exceeded or the payment of deductibles and copayments alone creates a major financial burden. In these programs the favored approach is "stop-loss" coverage, meant to take over on those rare occasions when care is so costly that traditional coverage is insufficient to protect a person or family from financially onerous out-of-pocket expenditures. Typically, therefore, stop-loss coverage presupposes the existence of other, basic coverage that is adequate for all but relatively rare devastating occurrences (Beam and McFadden, 1985, and Mehr and Gustafson, 1987).

That kind of stop-loss coverage, however, is not likely to meet the needs of families such as those just described, which have out-of-pocket health services expenditures that are high in relation to their incomes. Undoubtedly some of these families are the kind that, despite having insurance, were financially overwhelmed by a high-cost illness and would therefore definitely benefit from stop-loss coverage. The great majority, however, are more aptly described as medically indigent and low-income uninsured families that need very basic health care coverage to avoid the heavy financial burden almost any medical care expenditure would impose on them. In fact, much of the catastrophic coverage such families need is indistinguishable from the programs now being proposed and considered for the medically indigent. (See, for example, Mulstein, 1984; Farley, 1985; Monheit et al., 1985; and Employee Benefit Research Institute, 1987.)

Yet in the few documented instances where a catastrophic coverage program has served such medically indigent persons, it has done so unintentionally. According to one state-by-state survey, all three state catastrophic health programs that were in operation in early 1984—those in Alaska, Maine, and Rhode Island—had been restructured in preceding years "to prevent them from serving as health insurance programs for indigents" (Desonia and King, 1985). Among other changes, the three programs had imposed large deductibles to preclude covering relatively small expenditures, even when these expenditures represent a ruinous financial burden for a low-income family with no other health care coverage.

Single-Dollar Limits—An additional characteristic of stop-loss coverage and of other types of catastrophic proposals that limits their usefulness for those who have financially catastrophic expenditures is the tendency to specify eligibility for coverage in terms of a single-dollar amount.

The Long-Ribicoff* catastrophic insurance bill of 1979 is typical in that respect. It would have provided coverage to everyone whose out-of-pocket health care expenditures were greater than $2,000 (in 1979 dollars) during a year's time.

Similarly, the measure passed by the Senate in October 1987 (S. 1127) specifies that Medicare beneficiaries would be eligible for catastrophic coverage in 1988 once their out-of-pocket expenditures exceed $1,850 for that year. Such single-dollar limits, however, do not take into account differences in ability to pay, and therefore coverage is provided to some who do not need it while it is denied to others who do. For example, an expense of $1,850 is not likely to be financially catastrophic for individuals or families with incomes over $40,000. Providing coverage to them at that level, therefore, is at least premature and could prove altogether unnecessary. By contrast, the same single-dollar limit will fail to extend timely coverage to those for whom even relatively small amounts such as $500 already represent a financially catastrophic expenditure because their financial resources are so severely limited.

The Focus on Acute Care—Another limitation of most past catastrophic coverage proposals and programs is their scope of coverage, which is typically restricted to acute-care services. The measure passed by the Senate follows that tradition. The out-of-pocket expenses counted toward the cap take into account only the deductibles, coinsurance,

---

*Editor's note: Former Senators Russell Long (D-LA) and Abraham Ribicoff (D-CN).

and other amounts paid for physician and hospital services that are covered by Medicare. The catastrophic coverage, in turn, is limited to such services. Out-of-pocket amounts spent on services such as basic nursing home care that are not covered by Medicare are not counted toward eligibility nor are those services covered under the catastrophic measure. Yet nursing home and other long-term care expenditures account for much of the risk that the elderly face of incurring catastrophic health expenditures (U.S. Congress, 1984, 1985).

Combining a focus on acute-care services with a stop-loss approach, as most proposals do, has further implications, given the characteristics of high-cost hospitalizations, for which such proposals are most directly intended.

Consequences of Improved Coverage of High-Cost Hospitalizations— The most recent description of the characteristics of high-cost hospitalizations is based on an analysis of patients discharged from 54 hospitals in Maryland during 1981 (Berki et al.,1983).[1] In this analysis, a person was considered to be a high-cost case if his or her total hospital charges exceeded $7,500 for the 1981 calendar year.

Overall, several categories of discharges or patients emerged as particularly likely to be high-cost cases: those discharged dead; those with multiple discharges; those over 55 years of age; newborns with problems of immaturity; patients in diagnosis-related groups (DRGs) involving cardiac surgery (especially coronary bypass), surgery on joints, and surgery related to cancers. In some DRGs, all or nearly all discharges were high-cost: valve surgery on heart (DRGs 104 and 105), coronary bypass (DRGs 106 and 107), and kidney transplant (DRG 302). It was also found that a disproportionate number of high-cost cases were discharged from teaching hospitals with over 400 beds.

In light of these findings, it would appear that catastrophic health care coverage programs directed at high-cost hospitalizations—because they focus on acute care and take a stop-loss approach—risk incurring important, presumably unintended consequences. The more complete coverage they would afford all high-cost acute care cases would improve the financing for procedures that, in addition to being high-cost, are controversial, such as coronary bypass surgery, a costly operation believed by some to be performed more often than appro-

---

[1]As part of the same study, a parallel analysis was performed using data from a set of hospitals that subscribe to the services offered by the Commission of Professional and Hospital Activities; it yielded results very similar to those described in the text.

priate (Kolata, 1983) and some organ transplants, whose high cost has been questioned given the uncertain benefits that result from them.

Similarly, the greater coverage that these catastrophic programs would provide for high-cost care for premature newborns and the terminally ill may raise more forcefully complex ethical issues about the quality and value of life and death and require the explicit resolution of very perplexing resource allocation problems. Another consequence of better coverage may be to increase the flow of resources to the larger teaching hospitals that account for a disproportionate share of high-cost cases, at a time when the higher costs associated with such hospitals are being questioned.

The Focus on High-Cost Diseases—The longstanding tendency to equate high-cost cases with financially catastrophic ones has resulted in periodic calls for catastrophic coverage programs focused on illnesses requiring very expensive treatment. This approach proved successful for one of these high-cost illnesses, end-stage renal disease (ESRD), when in 1973 the Medicare program began covering virtually everyone with ESRD.

Although subsequent attempts to provide similar coverage for hemophilia and end-stage heart disease proved unsuccessful, and, in fact, led to the questioning of such a disease-by-disease approach (Institute of Medicine, 1973), there has been renewed interest in illness-specific coverage with the epidemic spread of acquired immunodeficiency syndrome (AIDS).[2]

It is still uncertain what the exact costs of AIDS are, but it is quite clear that it is a high-cost illness (Sisk, 1987). Nevertheless, a blanket provision of public coverage for everyone who suffers from AIDS— or from any other high-cost disease or condition—whatever its other attributes, is both too narrow and too indiscriminate as a form of catastrophic coverage. Such an approach inevitably covers some who do not need it—because they have other coverage—while it covers others sooner than they require it (before their other coverage has been exhausted), and it fails to cover at all the many financially catastrophic cases that are not the result of the target illness or illnesses.

---

[2]For example, interest in illness-specific coverage is reflected in the provisions of H. R. 2880, introduced in 1983, under which Medicare would cover virtually all AIDS cases.

29

Developing and Adopting a New Definition: Initial Hurdles

To formulate a generally consistent and satisfactory definition of catastrophic health expenditures, a number of issues must be resolved, many of them relatively technical and abstruse. But even before such issues can be meaningfully addressed, two major hurdles must be overcome: the attitudes that bolster stop-loss approaches and the ever-present concern with cost containment.

Attitudes that Bolster Stop-Loss Approaches—It is unlikely that for the past several decades catastrophic health coverage programs have relied so consistently on stop-less approaches merely out of inattention to definitional consistency. More likely the choice was a deliberate one, reflecting an inclination to cover only the segment of the population that, although it has basic health insurance, is still financially vulnerable when faced with high-cost illnesses. Put in starker terms, the intended beneficiaries are mostly the members of the middle and upper classes who, although sufficiently provident and with the necessary resources to have obtained health insurance, are still at some risk. The goal of most catastrophic proposals and programs is to protect this group against the much-feared instances where the extensive need for health services, in addition to all its other consequences, results in out-of-pocket costs that threaten the financial stability of the family.

As was mentioned, the structure and development of several state catastrophic coverage programs reflects an explicit desire to cover such people, coupled with efforts not to cover the poor and medically indigent through the same mechanism. Maine's Catastrophic Illness Program (CIP), for example, is notable for *not* having been set up as a stop-loss program. Originally, to qualify for it a person had to have incurred out-of-pocket health expenditures equal to 20 percent of net income plus 10 percent of net worth and $1,000.

Given such criteria, the great majority of those who qualified for the program were the poor and the uninsured; most of them were not high-cost cases. Thus, during the first five years of the program's operation (1975 to 1980), the average amount paid per recipient was $2,110 and 95 percent of claims were for amounts under $1,000. This was an unintended and unwelcome result, as noted in an independent evaluation of the CIP's first five years:

> The legislature intended the program for persons with extraordinary medical expenses whose private health insurance benefits were not ad-

equate to cover their expenses, leaving them vulnerable to a loss of their assets (house, car, etc.). However, most of the beneficiaries of the program were not among this group; it was the poor, the unemployed, the uninsured, and those without resources who were the primary beneficiaries of the Maine CIP during this time period (Deprez, 1983).

In an attempt to redirect the program toward those it meant to serve, and to curb rising costs, the Maine legislature raised the deductible from $1,000 to $7,000, effectively restricting coverage to those who are both financially catastrophic and high-cost cases. As noted earlier, other state catastrophic insurance programs were similarly restructured "to prevent them from serving as health insurance programs for indigents" (Desonia and King, 1985).

Given this rather clearly expressed preference to exclude the indigent and the uninsured, arguing for a definition of catastrophic expenditures that both applies to everyone and relates to ability to pay may be futile without first considering what may account for the preference. One immediate response is to attribute this preference to a lack of compassion for people who are less well-off; if that is indeed the case, calls for internally consistent definitions are apt to fall on deaf ears.

There is, however, the possibility that the attitudes spring from— or at least are reinforced by—misconceptions that could be dispelled by examining their basic premises and by citing known facts. Among potential misconceptions, two are especially likely: the view that, because the poor have so little money, the smallest health expense can qualify as financially catastrophic when in reality it is not; and the belief that there already are programs to provide health care for the poor.

According to the first assertion, a health expenditure is not truly catastrophic unless it is also a large one. In terms of the classification described at the outset, this is equivalent to restricting the definition of financially catastrophic cases to the area of overlap between the catastrophic and high-cost categories, thereby leaving out all the cases that are financially catastrophic but not high-cost (see chart III.1). In other words, this eliminates cases in which a relatively small expenditure proves to be beyond the affected person's or family's ability to pay, presumably because of severely limited resources. Yet in such cases, because disposable income is apt to be so limited—there is little or no ability to withstand any expenses beyond the barest necessities—the need for protection is, if anything, more pressing than it is for the traditional targets of catastrophic programs, those who are financially catastrophic cases because they have high-cost expenditures.

As for the second assertion, that there are already programs to provide coverage for the poor, it is at best only partly correct and has become increasingly less so over the past several years. It is now estimated that close to 60 percent of the nonelderly population that is below the federal poverty standard has neither Medicaid nor any other health coverage. This is an increase from what it was earlier in the decade (Chollet, 1987; Mulstein, 1984; and Farley, 1985). In addition, many of the providers of last resort for such people, particularly city and county hospitals, have closed their doors during the last 10 years, leaving the medically indigent at the mercy of institutions that themselves are increasingly unable or unwilling to provide charity care. The growing attention to "indigent care" attests to how much worse this problem has become. It is difficult, therefore, to make a convincing case for excluding the poor from catastrophic coverage programs by claiming that they are already covered by other, special programs such as Medicaid. Recent trends actually support the opposite argument.

Concern with Cost Containment—Cost containment is another general concern that influences how catastrophic programs define who is and is not eligible. The long-standing practice of excluding from catastrophic and other types of coverage expenditures for services such as long-term care—particularly nursing home care—outpatient drugs, and mental health is attributable not so much to confusion over definitions as to fears that the costs of covering these kinds of services could easily become unmanageable. In the best tradition of past proposals for catastrophic coverage, all of the recent proposals for Medicare beneficiaries have focused on expenditures for acute hospital and physician services, even though the proportion of beneficiaries who currently exceed Medicare's coverage limit on hospitalizations is very small, less than 0.2 percent in any given year (Gornick et al., 1983).

On the other hand, because most nursing home and other long-term care expenditures are currently not covered by Medicare, nearly 3 million elderly persons who need such care are at risk of incurring financially catastrophic expenditures (U.S. Congress, 1985). Only after they reach almost total impoverishment can they expect some relief, and then not from Medicare but from the Medicaid program. As long as expenditures for nursing home care are not covered by a catastrophic program for the elderly, those who need this care will continue to be subjected to the very financial difficulties and

32

indignities from which the traditional stop-loss approach has sought to shield people.

A further paradox is that, to the extent that cost-containment considerations dictate a narrow focus for catastrophic programs, they actually increase the potential for still higher costs: the continued emphasis on acute care is likely to channel more resources to the larger teaching hospitals that provide most of the high-cost services and, more generally, to promote the use of costly high-technology services in lieu of long-term care, all of which is likely to result in higher total expenditures for care with few prospects of a commensurate gain in total benefits.

Addressing the Definitional Issues Proper

Even if a broad social consensus is forged to direct catastrophic programs at everyone whose health care expenditures exceed his or her ability to pay—in other words, at all financially catastrophic cases—with neither ideological nor cost-containment considerations allowed to distort how a catastrophic case is defined, a number of important definitional issues would still need to be resolved. The two most basic are how to specify and measure "ability to pay" and what exactly a "health care expenditure" ought to encompass.

Defining Ability to Pay—One's ability to pay for health care services obviously depends on one's total resources. An initial question in identifying those resources is *whose* resources are to be considered: those of the individual who incurred the health care expenditures or those of a broader group of people associated with the person, typically the family of that individual.

• Individual versus Family. The resources generally considered to be available to pay for health care more often than not are pooled at the level of the nuclear family. Health care coverage, whether in the form of private insurance or that of public programs, is often extended to the principal beneficiary's spouse and minor children. Similarly, income and savings are typically shared within the nuclear family, especially in the context of dealing with unusually burdensome health care expenditures.

However, whereas it may be widely acceptable to postulate a shared responsibility for health care expenditures within the prototypical nuclear family that consists of a married couple and its minor children, definitions that encompass other family members—the extended family—are likely to prove much more controversial. Although there are many instances of members of an extended family helping one another pay for health care bills, there has never been much enthusiasm for schemes that take such help for granted. Grandparents would not want to be financially liable for their grandchildren's health care bills even though many are inclined to help financially if a costly illness does strike. Similarly, measures that hold adult children financially responsible for even a portion of their parents' health care, with public assistance covering the rest, are invariably unpopular.

Even within the nuclear family, the sharing of this kind of financial responsibility has been recognized to have its limits. For example, the Medicare Catastrophic Coverage Act of 1988 includes a provision that will protect the living standard of the spouse of an elderly person whose institutionalization in a nursing home ends up being covered by Medicaid.

Separation, divorce, and remarriage lead to family configurations and relations that are quite different from and usually more complex than implied by the model of the nuclear family. That, however, does not necessarily translate into further difficulties in determining who should pay for whose care, since such matters usually have been worked out quite formally and are spelled out in legal documents associated with divorce, adoption, and marriage. But when that is not the case, the fashioning of fair and acceptable rules of responsibility for health care expenditures presents a difficult challenge.

• Specification of Resources. The resources considered available for paying for care—and therefore the ones that determine ability to pay—are of three types: third-party health care coverage; income from all sources; and wealth, consisting of all accumulated assets.

By specifying eligibility thresholds in terms of out-of-pocket health expenditures, virtually all catastrophic programs and proposals take into account implicitly, and often explicitly as well, health insurance, public program payments for health care, and other forms of third-party payment.

Catastrophic programs that take a purely stop-loss approach usually have a threshold that is specified in terms of a single-dollar amount, and thus do not consider either income or assets. Most other programs, however, do take income into account and determine eligibility by comparing out-of-pocket expenditures to income. The relation between the two is specified in terms that range from very simple to relatively complex. At one end is Feldstein's Major Risk Insurance Proposal, which simply sets the threshold at 10 percent of income (Feldstein, 1971). By contrast, the Martin bill (H.R. 6405), introduced in 1980, divided the population into three income groups and stipulated for them a graduated set of flat deductibles plus a percentage of income; for example, families with incomes below $4,000 are subject only to a simple $300 deductible, whereas those with incomes above $10,000 must meet a $1,500 deductible plus 20 percent of any income they have above $10,000.

Few catastrophic programs consider assets. Between 1981 and 1984, when it was discontinued, Maine's CIP was among the few with a threshold that included, in addition to 30 percent of net income, 10 percent of "net worth" over $20,000. Net worth was defined as the market value of all real and personal property, including all cashable and noncashable assets, minus encumbrances and liabilities (Desonia and King, 1985).

How income and assets are specified and measured, and what portion of them is considered available to pay for care in catastrophic coverage programs, ultimately represents an expression of society's view of how much a person's or a family's standard of living should be allowed to deteriorate because of health care expenditures. It also reflects how equitably and universally help is to be extended to all members of society. In this context, the following considerations have special saliency:

1. Illness can substantially reduce the income of a family, either because the one who is ill is a wage earner or because looking after the person who is ill reduces the capacity of one or more wage earners in the family to earn income. It is therefore important to make determinations of income levels that correspond to the period during which health care expenditures are being accumulated, rather than for some prior period.

2. As some proposals implicitly acknowledge, the percentage of a person's or a family's income and assets that can be devoted to health care without creating undue financial stain is apt to vary across income levels: all else being equal, the lower the income, the more of this income is likely to be spent on necessities, leaving little or nothing for nonrecurring and unpredictable items such as care for acute illnesses.

3. Even within the same income group, there can be substantial differences in ability to pay for health care because of variation in obligations that themselves derive from differences in family size, general cost of living in the community, and availability of and access to necessities such as housing, transportation, and child care services.

4. The inclusion of any assets in the computation of ability to pay for care is seen by many as penalizing those who have been thrifty and provident. It is argued further that in the long run this may, if not encourage profligacy, at least discourage savings. The inclusion

of nonliquid assets in the computation presents additional difficulties, particularly if one's home and automobile are included. Having to sell off assets that represent basic shelter and transportation can greatly add to the disruptions that illness already engenders. On the other hand, those who upon retirement sell their homes and become renters would see it as inequitable if the proceeds from their home were considered available to pay for health care whereas that money would have been protected had they not sold their home.

Finally, it should be noted that catastrophic health programs have approached the determination of ability to pay differently from our tax system and public assistance programs. Medicaid, for example, takes into account the differences in obligations represented by family size and it also considers assets such as bank accounts and life insurance. This is not to say that Medicaid or our tax system should necessarily serve as the models for catastrophic programs, but the experience with both is instructive. If nothing else, it suggests how difficult it is to find a satisfactory definition of ability to pay even when the objectives being pursued are reasonably clear, as in the case of taxation (Musgrave and Musgrave, 1973).

Inclusiveness of Expenditures—Earlier I made a case for including expenditures for long-term care in the definition of health care expenditures rather than consistently excluding them, as has been done in response to cost-containment and other concerns. I pointed out that such an exclusion runs counter to the basic goal of catastrophic programs, that of covering health care expenditures that exceed a person's or family's ability to pay. Ultimately, it does not matter whether expenditures are for long-term care, mental health services, prescription drugs, or some other form of health care. The financial impact on individuals and families is the same. Therefore, for a catastrophic program to achieve its fundamental goal, eligibility and coverage must be specified in terms of a broad definition of health care expenditures.

Still, it must be established explicitly just how all-encompassing the definition of health care expenditures ought to be, particularly for expenditures that many regard to be discretionary and therefore not appropriate for coverage by catastrophic programs. This includes orthodontia, cosmetic surgery, certain kinds of psychotherapy, fertility-related services, and even care received from high-priced providers whose services include many nonessential amenities.

Another category of expenditures that some would argue are not properly *health care* expenditures are those that, although occasioned by illness or disability, are largely or totally for nonhealth care services, being mostly for what are more appropriately classified as either custodial or social services. This argument is most frequently directed at certain long-term services such as basic nursing home care and adult day care, in which the health care component can be quite small. Ultimately, the issue is how much weight should be placed, in classifying an expenditure, on the health care content of the services and the training of those who provide them, as opposed to the nature of the situation that led to the provision of the services, specifically whether it is related to an illness or disability or, instead, to a social need, such as the lack of a family to look after a frail but not disabled or ill elderly person.

Toward a Working Definition

Given all the foregoing, how should we proceed in formulating a definition of catastrophic health expenditures, if this definition is to provide the basis for a meaningful and effective catastrophic coverage program? Whatever the specific strategy adopted, it is more likely to produce the desired results if it takes into consideration and ultimately reflects relevant social goals and values; takes proper account of the nature of health care; and acknowledges practical problems, particularly the availability of the requisite information and the costs of gathering it.

Social Values and Goals—I have argued that a definition of financially catastrophic expenditures will have both logical consistency and intuitive appeal on its side if it is based on the relation between health care expenditures and the ability to pay for them and if the size of the total amount expended is not a factor. However, such a definition inevitably applies to most health care expenses incurred by the poor and uninsured, and it may be resisted for that reason by those who conceive of catastrophic coverage as a stop-loss program to protect people who already have coverage for all but the most high-cost occurrences. This alternative, and in a sense truncated, definition is bound to be proposed and therefore needs to be considered. The chief objection to it is likely to be its inequity, particularly given the worsening prospects for coverage faced by the medically indigent, whom it is designed to exclude.

This suggests that, more generally, a definition of financially catastrophic expenditures, to be meaningful and acceptable, must reflect the nature and extent of our society's fundamental commitment to shielding people from the financial burdens imposed by health care expenditures and to do so equitably. The same applies to the more specific definition of ability to pay: basic values ought to inform explicitly our decision about how much we are willing to let a person's standard of living deteriorate before relief is provided. Accomplishing this is no easy task, because in essence it requires that an appropriate balance be struck between social responsibility and individual responsibility for health care expenditures.

The Nature of Health Care and Illness—The long-standing emphasis of catastrophic coverage programs on acute care services, particularly in terms of hospital care, reflects in large part the actuary's view of hospitalizations as meeting the criteria for an insurable risk reasonably well, in contrast to nursing home care and care for most mental illnesses, which are seen as quite far from meeting these insurability criteria. The resulting tendency to exclude such services from coverage is now reinforced by pervasive cost-containment concerns.

Yet illnesses and the cost of caring for them know no actuarial or fiscal barriers. A person who is financially ruined by expenditures for long-term care is neither more or less ruined than if the expenditures had been for hospital care. The need for protection is the same and programs that distinguish between the two types of expenditures do not alter this basic equivalence. Making the distinction actually sets up perverse incentives. For example, it encourages providing hospital care to someone who needs long-term care, because the first is covered but the other is not. The result is a dysfunctional and ultimately more expensive substitution that both violates the integrity of the medical care process (Donabedian, 1976) and at some level even works at cross purposes with the goal of cost-containment. It is therefore important to address directly the need for coverage for *all* illnesses and conditions, which, as the earlier discussion on defining health care expenditures clearly suggests, is yet another difficult task. But it is also a key one.

Practical Problems—Even if there is wide consensus on a definition of financially catastrophic expenditures that is logically consistent and responsive to actual needs for health care, there can still be practical problems that, along with the specter of unintended consequences, require modifications or simplifications that would otherwise be considered undesirable.

For example, seemingly reasonable eligibility thresholds may have to be altered or other actions taken if it appears that they may be low enough to induce some people to do away with their current health insurance and use the catastrophic program as their only coverage, where the catastrophic threshold becomes their deductible. One obvious solution to this problem is to make eligibility for the catastrophic program contingent on having prescribed levels of other coverage. But that leads to prescriptions of minimum coverage levels, which in turn raises the issue of how various groups in the population might obtain such coverage, thus broadening the scope and increasing the difficulty of the task even further.[3]

A potentially more intractable problem is the impracticality of making accurate assessments of a family's health care expenditures, health insurance coverage, income, and assets. This may not only be difficult and time-consuming, but it may be resisted by the potential beneficiaries themselves, on the grounds that some of these inquiries are demeaning and an invasion of privacy. Part of the appeal of single-dollar eligibility thresholds is that they avoid such problems, not to mention the considerable difficulties involved in deciding how to measure income and other resources and what portion of each ought to be deemed available for medical payments.

What Can Be Expected?

The difficulties, practical and conceptual, are indeed great, and no perfect definition of financially catastrophic expenditures is ever likely to emerge that will help us set up the perfect catastrophic coverage program. But great progress can be made if we identify and acknowledge the shortcomings of most of the definitions we now have. This would set the stage for systematically improving them, by taking advantage of the kind of conceptual and definitional distinctions and relations that have been described here and by recognizing explicitly the role of social values and goals in this kind of undertaking.

References

Beam, B.T., Jr., and J.J. McFadden. *Employee Benefits.* Homewood, IL: Richard D. Irwin, 1985.

Berki, S.E., L. Wyszewianski, and P.A. Gimotty. *High Cost Illness among Hospitalized Patients.* Report to the U.S. Department of Health

---

[3]Eligibility rules for Rhode Island's catastrophic health insurance program provide substantial incentives for people to be covered by "qualified" health insurance plans. (See Desonia and King, 1985.)

and Human Services, National Center for Health Services Research. Washington, DC: U.S. Government Printing Office, 1983. (NTIS no. PB84-239110.

Chollet, D.J. "Financing Indigent Health Care." In F.B. McArdle, ed. *The Changing Health Care Market*. Washington, DC: Employee Benefit Research Institute, 1987.

Deprez, R.D.; B. Curran; and M.S. Spindler. *A Study of Maine's Catastrophic Illness Program, 1975-1980*. Augusta, ME: Medical Care Development, Inc., 1983.

Desonia, R.A., and K.M. King. *State Programs of Assistance for the Medically Indigent*. Intergovernmental Health Policy Project. Washington, DC: George Washington University, 1985.

Donabedian, A. *Benefits in Medical Care Programs*. Cambridge MA: Harvard University Press, 1976.

Employee Benefit Research Institute. "Public Options to Expand Health Insurance Coverage Among the Nonelderly Population."*EBRI Issue Brief* 67 (June 1987).

Farley, P.J. "Who Are the Underinsured?" *Milbank Memorial Fund Quarterly* 63 (Fall 1985): 476.

Feldstein, M.S. "A New Approach to National Health Insurance." *The Public Interest* 23 (Spring 1971): 251–280.

Gornick, M.; J. Beebee; and R. Prihoda. "Options for Change Under Medicare: Impact of a Cap on Catastrophic Illness Expense." *Health Care Financing Review* 5 (Fall 1983): 33–43.

Institute of Medicine. *Disease by Disease Toward National Health Insurance?* Washington, DC: National Academy of Sciences, 1973.

Kasper, J.A.; R. Anderson; and C. Brown. *The Financial Impact of Catastrophic Illness as Measured in the CHAS-NORCA National Survey*. Chicago, IL: University of Chicago, 1975.

Kolata, G. "Some Bypass Surgery Unnecessary." *Science* 222 (November 11, 1983): 605.

Mehr, R.I., and S.G. Gustafson. *Life Insurance: Theory and Practice*. Plano, TX: Business Publications, 1987.

Monheit, A.C.; M.M. Hagan; M.L. Berk; and P.J. Farley. "The Employed Uninsured and the Role of Public Policy." *Inquiry* 22 (Winter 1985): 348.

Mulstein, S. "The Uninsured and the Financing of Uncompensated Care: Scope, Costs, and Policy Options." *Inquiry* 21 (Fall 1984): 214.

Musgrave, R.A., and P.B. Musgrave. *Public Finance in Theory and in Practice*. New York: McGraw-Hill, 1973.

Sisk, J.E. "The Cost of AIDS." *Health Affairs* 6 (Summer 1987): 5–21.

U.S. Congress. House. Select Committee on Aging. *America's Elderly at Risk*. Washington, DC: U.S. Government Printing Office, 1985.

U.S. Congress. Senate. Special Committee on Aging. *Medicare and the Health Costs of Older Americans: The Extent and Effects of Cost Sharing*. Washington, DC: U.S. Government Printing Office, 1984.

Van Ellet, T. *State Comprehensive and Catastrophic Health Insurance Programs: An Overview*. Intergovernmental Health Policy Project. Washington, DC: George Washington University, 1981.

Wyszewianski, L. "Financially Catastrophic and High-Cost Cases: Definitions, Distinctions, and Their Implications for Policy Formulation." *Inquiry* 23 (Winter 1986): 382–394.

Wyszewianski, L. "Families with Catastrophic Health Care Expenditures." *Health Services Research* 21 (December 1986): 617–634.

IV. Catastrophic Health Care Costs: Who Is at Risk?

PAPER BY DEBORAH CHOLLET AND CHARLES BETLEY

Introduction

Nearly three-quarters of the nonelderly population have private health insurance coverage, and more than two-thirds are covered by employer-provided group health plans. Nevertheless, many people—including some with insurance coverage—remain at risk for uninsured catastrophic health care costs. People with individually purchased or employer-sponsored private insurance, or with coverage from public programs like Medicaid, may not be fully covered for all types of health care expenses. For people without insurance coverage, any major illness can result in a catastrophic level of health care expense.

To assess uninsured risk among the general population, a definition of catastrophic expenses must be developed. This paper examines alternative definitions of catastrophic expense and their implications for the size and distribution of the nonelderly population likely to incur uninsured catastrophic expenses; examines the relationship between types of insurance coverage and levels of catastrophic expenses; and discusses public policy concerns related to two high-risk populations—chronically or severely ill children and acquired immune deficiency syndrome (AIDS) victims.

Defining Catastrophic Health Care Costs

Catastrophic levels of health care expenses can be defined absolutely (as uninsured expenses exceeding an absolute dollar threshold) or relatively (as uninsured expenses exceeding some percentage of family income). Alternative definitions of catastrophic health care costs can lead to different perceptions about the size and characteristics of the populations most vulnerable to incurring catastrophic expenses.

Most private insurers define catastrophic health care expenses in terms of an absolute dollar amount. Private insurance limits on both beneficiary out-of-pocket expenses and plan liability defined as dollar amounts are common. Only 4 percent of workers who participate in

43

medium or large employer plans have limits on participant cost sharing defined relative to their earnings.

An absolute-dollar definition of catastrophic health care expenses, however, fails to account for differences among families' ability to finance care. Consequently, some researchers have argued that a more appropriate definition is one that relates uninsured expenses to family income (Wyszewianski, pp. 23–26). By such a definition, however, very low-income families may find virtually any level of uninsured medical expense catastrophic—including relatively modest expenses for routine medical care.

In its report on catastrophic health care financing, the U.S. Department of Health and Human Services (HHS) has suggested that the discussion of financing catastrophic health care expenses should distinguish between the issues of financing routine health care for the low-income population and financing health care that would represent a catastrophic expense for most families (HHS, 1986). The HHS report proposes a composite definition for uninsured catastrophic expense: uninsured expenses that exceed both an absolute dollar amount (e.g., $2,200) and, above that, a percentage of family income (e.g., 10 percent). The HHS definition would focus on improbably high health care expenditures (avoiding the discussion of routine care that may be financially catastrophic for low-income families), but retain some reference to families' ability to pay.

As a feature of either private or public health insurance arrangements, however, this type of definition is administratively complex. Employer health insurance plans only rarely include coverage provisions related to earnings, and never relate coverage to family income. Although state Medicaid programs determine monthly eligibility in part on the basis of family income (and, in some states, family income after health care expenses are subtracted), this process of "means testing" involves substantial administrative cost for Medicaid and/or for means-tested cash assistance programs that confer Medicaid eligibility.

How the Definition of Catastrophic Expenses Determines Who Is at Risk

How catastrophic costs are defined shapes who is perceived to be at risk of incurring catastrophic expenses. By virtually any definition, however, families in poverty are more likely to have catastrophic levels of uninsured health care expenses than nonpoor families. If the catastrophic costs are defined as uninsured costs above some percentage of family income, poor families are much more likely than nonpoor families to incur catastrophic expenses. If the catastrophic threshold is defined as a fixed dollar level of uninsured expense, the difference between poor and nonpoor families in their probabilities of incurring catastrophic expenses narrows. In 1977, among people in families that incurred uninsured health care expenses equal to 20 percent or more of family income, 66.1 percent were poor. Among families with uninsured health care expenses above $2,200 (in 1987 dollars), 15.2 percent were poor (table IV.1). By comparison, among the population as a whole, 11.6 percent of all persons and 9.3 percent of families were poor in 1977.

The definition of catastrophic expenses also influences the relative effects of noncoverage and underinsurance on the likelihood of incurring uninsured, catastrophic health care expenses. In 1985, about 37 million nonelderly people (17 percent of the population under age 65) lacked health insurance coverage from any public or private source (Employee Benefit Research Institute, 1987).

Table IV.2 shows the proportion of individuals in 1980 living in families that experienced catastrophic health care expenses (using alternative definitions), with different sources of insurance coverage. These estimates differ from those presented in table IV.1 primarily because they refer to only the nonelderly population and count individuals rather than families.

TABLE IV.1
Percentage of Families with Uninsured Catastrophic Health Care Expenses by Various Thresholds of Catastrophic Expense and Percentage in Poverty, 1977[a]

Threshold of Catastrophic Expense	Percentage of All Families with Uninsured Catastrophic Expenses	Percentage of Families with These Uninsured Catastrophic Expenses That Are in Poverty
$2,200 or more[b]	4.9%	15.2%
5 percent of family income	19.9	31.5
10 percent of family income	9.6	47.5
20 percent of family income	4.3	66.1

Sources: U.S. Department of Health and Human Services, *Catastrophic Illness Expenses, Report to the President* (Washington, DC: U.S. Government Printing Office, 1986), technical chapter 2, table 2-2A; and Leon Wyszewianski, "Families with Catastrophic Health Care Expenditures," *Health Services Research* 21 (December 1986), tables 2–4.
[a]Data include both elderly and nonelderly families.
[b]In 1987 dollars.

TABLE IV.2
Percentage of Nonelderly People in Families with Health Insurance Coverage Experiencing Various Levels of Uninsured Catastrophic Expenditures, 1980

Covered Population:	Out-of-Pocket Expenditures in Excess of							
	$1,000[a]	$2,000[a]	$3,500[a]	$4,000[a]	$7,000[a]	5% of family income	10% of family income	20% of family income
Total	28.4%	11.1%	3.9%	2.8%	0.2%	11.0%	3.7%	2.1%
Total insured	28.8	11.1	3.9	2.8	0.7	10.3	4.3	1.8
Private insurance employer-paid	29.9	11.0	3.8	2.8	0.7	8.0	3.0	1.1
individual	34.6	15.1	5.1	3.4	0.7	17.2	7.7	3.2
Public insurance	17.8	6.6	2.5	2.1	0.5	13.2	6.5	3.0
Uninsured	23.4	10.8	3.9	3.1	0.7	18.8	9.3	5.2

Source: EBRI tabulations of the National Medical Care Utilization and Expenditure Survey public use data tape, U.S. Department of Health and Human Services, National Center for Health Statistics, 1980.

[a]In 1986 dollars.

Paradoxically, the population with individual, private insurance coverage is more likely than the uninsured population to incur catastrophic expenses, if catastrophic expenses are defined in terms of a dollar threshold of uninsured spending. In 1980, 15 percent of the population with private, individual coverage lived in families that incurred uninsured expenses of $2,000 or more (in 1986 dollars), compared to less than 11 percent of the uninsured population.

If catastrophic expenses are defined relative to income, however, the uninsured population is more likely than the individually insured population to incur uninsured catastrophic expenses. In 1980, 9.3 percent of the uninsured population were in families that spent 10 percent or more of their family income for health care, compared to nearly 8 percent of the population with individual private coverage. More than five percent of the uninsured lived in families that incurred catastrophic health care expenses equal to 20 percent or more of family income, compared to 3 percent of those with individual private insurance.

By most measures of catastrophic expense, the population with employer-based insurance coverage is less likely to have uninsured catastrophic expenses than either the individually insured or uninsured populations. In 1980, 11 percent of the nonelderly population insured by employers had uninsured health care expenses of $2,000 or more, compared to 15.1 percent of nonelderly people with individual private coverage. Three percent of the employer-insured population lived in families with uninsured health care expenses equal to 10 percent or more of family income, compared to 9.3 percent of the uninsured population.

Differences in the likelihood of incurring catastrophic expenses among people with different sources of insurance coverage may be explained by differences in coverage, behavior, and access to health care services. Employer group plans may cover more services and pay for a greater proportion of the costs than do private, individual insurance plans, reducing the likelihood of uninsured catastrophic expenses among people with employer-based coverage. Higher out-of-pocket spending by the population with private, individual coverage compared with that by the uninsured population may be a consequence of greater access to care among people with insurance. It may also reflect adverse selection (i.e., the greater likelihood that people will purchase insurance coverage if they expect to use health care services). As a result, people with individual private insurance may use more health care than the uninsured and may incur greater out-of-pocket expenses not covered by their insurance plans.

The generally lower family income of publicly insured people may largely explain the relatively high rate of their catastrophic expenditures relative to income. Health care expenses that might not be insured by public plans (including dental care, vision care, and prescription drugs) may pose catastrophic expenses (relative to income) for very low-income families. States may also limit the scope and duration of services covered by Medicaid. For example, 17 states limit the duration of hospital stays for which Medicaid will pay.[1] The cost of a longer stay may be billed to the patient (potentially adding to a hospital's bad debt), or it may be directly financed by the hospital as charity care.

The likelihood of incurring catastrophic expenses among people with different insurance arrangements also varies with the types of insurance coverage held by people that incur catastrophic expenses (table IV.3). If uninsured catastrophic expenses are defined as incurred expenses above a dollar threshold, the distribution of insurance coverage among the population with catastrophic expenses is about the same as that among the population as a whole. That is, the proportion of people with catastrophic expenses (relative to a dollar threshold) who are covered by employer-based plans (63 to 68 percent) is similar to the proportion of people with employer coverage among the population as a whole (64.2 percent). However, if catastrophic expenses are defined as uninsured expenses equal to 20 percent or more of family income, the uninsured population (22 percent) and the population with coverage from public plans (28.4 percent) are disproportionately large segments of the population that incurs catastrophic costs (table IV.3).

The rate of catastrophic expenses that occurs among the population, however, generally understates the proportion of the population that is at risk for catastrophic health care expenses. That is, many people who do not actually experience catastrophic events nonetheless have some risk of experiencing such an event. If risk is defined as a one percent chance of spending more than $2,100 (in 1986 dollars) on health care during the year, one estimate (based on 1977 data) places 18 percent of the total population (including people over age 65) at risk for catastrophic health care expenses. If risk is defined as a one percent chance of spending more than 10 percent of family

---

[1]These states include: Alabama, Arkansas, Florida, Idaho, Illinois, Kentucky, Louisiana, Michigan, Mississippi, Ohio, Oklahoma, Oregon, South Carolina, Tennessee, Texas, Virginia, and West Virginia.

TABLE IV.3

Distribution of Insurance Coverage among Noninstitutionalized Persons under 65 Years Old in Families Experiencing Catastrophic Events, 1980 (in 1986 dollars)

Out-of-Pocket Expenditures in Excess of:	Uninsured	Insured			
		All sources public and private	Employer-paid private insurance	Private individual insurance not paid by employers	Public coverage[a]
$1,000	6.9%	93.1%	67.8%	20.8%	11.4%
$2,000	8.1	91.9	63.9	22.9	10.9
$3,500	8.3	91.7	63.5	22.5	12.0
$4,000	9.1	90.9	63.1	20.6	13.6
$7,000	8.0	92.0	68.4	16.3	12.6
5 percent of family income	13.0	87.0	49.3	25.9	17.8
10 percent of family income	17.3	82.7	38.8	26.7	23.8
20 percent of family income	22.0	78.0	30.6	26.2	28.4
All Persons	8.4	91.6	64.2	17.0	18.5

Source: EBRI tabulations of the National Medical Care Utilization and Expenditure Survey public use data tape, U.S. Department of Health and Human Services, National Center for Health Statistics, 1980.

[a]Public coverage category may include persons who also have private coverage, so columns may sum to greater than 100 percent.

income on health care, nearly 13 percent of the total population may be at risk of incurring catastrophic health care expenses (Farley, 1985).

Catastrophic Coverage in Employer Plans

Little is known about the specific sources of catastrophic health care costs for participants in employer plans. Employer plans vary in whether and how they limit plan liability and participants' liability for the costs of covered services. Whether the copayment features of employer health benefit plans or the plan limits are more responsible for the occurrence of catastrophic expenditures among the employer-insured population than are uncovered services is unknown.

Recent survey data on employer health benefit plans show that limits on out-of-pocket liabilities among employer-sponsored plans are common. A 1986 survey of medium and large employers (U.S. Department of Labor, 1987) found more than one-half of health plan participants had copayment provisions that limited their out-of-pocket expenses for covered services to $1,200 or less; about three-quarters had plans that limited out-of-pocket expenses for covered services to $2,000 or less. However, 19 percent of plan participants (approximately 4.1 million workers) had plans with no provision limiting their out-of-pocket expenses for covered services (table IV.4). Another survey in 1986 conducted for the Small Business Administration (ICF, Inc., 1987) found that small firms generally included higher out-of-pocket limits than larger firms. Of firms with more than 500 employees, 88 percent limited liabilities to less than $2,000, while 68 percent of firms with one to 24 employees limited liabilities to under $2,000 (table IV.5).

Federally qualified health maintenance organizations (HMOs) established under the Health Maintenance Organization Act of 1973 provide specific necessary medical services without regard to the frequency, duration, or extent of health services used. The 27.7 million persons enrolled in HMOs as of March 31, 1987 (InterStudy, 1987) are thus largely protected from catastrophic expenses arising from acute medical problems. However, HMOs may specifically exclude other services from coverage, such as long-term outpatient mental health benefits, or nursing home care, for which the enrollee would still remain liable.

Most employer-based major medical plans do not cover any expense for covered services that exceeds the plan maximum. In 1986, 73 percent of employees who participated in health plans offered by

TABLE IV.4
Percentage of Full-Time Workers in Medium and Large Establishments with an Employer-Sponsored Major Medical Plan, with Various Plan Provisions Related to Participant Cost, 1986

Plan Provision		Percentage of Participants
Plan deductible		
$50 or less		11%
$51 to $100		47
$101 to $150		16
$151 to $200		15
More than $200		6
No deductible		1
Based on earnings		4
Summary: less than $200		90
Plan coinsurance		
Health plan pays all expenses when covered expenses reach	Maximum participant coinsurance[a]	
$2,000	$400	
$4,000	$800	10%
$6,000	$1,200	22
$8,000	$1,600	30
$10,000	$2,000	6
More than $10,000	Greater than $2,000	9
		4
Coinsurance reduced or unchanged	Unlimited	19
Plan maximum		
Lifetime maximum		
$50,000 or less		4%
$50,001 to $100,000		2
$100,001 to $250,000		19
$250,001 to $500,000		18
Greater than $500,000		25
Lifetime and annual or disability maximum		5
Annual or disability maximum only		7
No maximum		20

(continued)

TABLE IV.4 (continued)

Plan Provision	Percentage of Participants
Summary	
Maximum greater than $100,000	82
Maximum greater than $250,000	63

Source: U.S. Department of Labor, Bureau of Labor Statistics, *Employee Benefits in Medium and Large Firms, 1986* (Washington, DC: U.S. Government Printing Office, 1987), tables 34–36.

[a]Assumes 80 percent copayment. In 1986, 86 percent of employees in medium and large establishments who participated in employer-sponsored major medical coverage had plans that paid 80 percent of the cost of covered services after the deductible.

medium and large firms had a lifetime maximum on annual benefits payable for covered services (including those with a lifetime and annual or disability maximum); 20 percent had plans that imposed no lifetime maximum, paying unlimited benefits for covered services (table IV.4). Aggregating workers with lifetime maximums over $100,000 and those without lifetime maximums in 1986, 82 percent of workers with employer coverage from larger establishments had plans that paid at least $100,000 for covered services after the participant paid the deductible and copayment; 63 percent participated in plans that paid $250,000 or more. The number of plan participants that reach plan limits on covered services and are, therefore, responsible for additional costs beyond the copayments is not known.

Services not covered by the health plan are also potentially catastrophic in their costs. Although employer plans universally provide coverage for inpatient and outpatient hospital care, which are generally the most expensive services, some services are not covered. For example, 29 percent of workers who participated in health benefit plans offered by larger firms did not have any plan coverage for nursing home care in 1986; 33 percent plans had that did not cover home health care (U.S. Department of Labor, 1987). Other services that employer plans commonly do not cover (e.g., vision and dental care) are typically less expensive than institutional care.

Special High-Risk Populations

Public policymakers have recently recognized the special health care financing problems of two particular groups: chronically ill children (particularly children who depend on technologically sophisticated medical equipment for survival), and people with AIDS or AIDS-Related Complex (ARC).

TABLE IV.5
Percentage Distribution of Employers with One Plan, by Maximum Annual Out-of-Pocket Provisions

Maximum Out-of-pocket Payment	All Plans	Number of Employees in Firm						
		1–24	25–99	100–499	500 or more	Less than 100	100 or more	Less than 500
$1–999	30%	27%	42%	39%	39%	30%	39%	30%
$1,000–1,999	40	41	39	34	49	41	36	40
$2,000–4,999	6	6	4	6	5	6	6	6
$5,000 and over	10	11	5	3	0	10	2	10
No limit	5	6	4	5	7	6	5	5
Not applicable	8	5	6	14	0	8	12	8
Total	100	100	100	100	100	100	100	100

Source: ICF, Inc., *Health Care Coverage and Costs in Small and Large Businesses*, prepared for the U.S. Small Business Administration, April 15, 1987.

Each year, an estimated 5 to 10 percent of children in the United States incur health care expenses that exceed $10,000 (U.S. Congress, 1987). The American Academy of Pediatrics (1987) estimates that approximately 421,000 children (0.6 percent of all children) had out-of-pocket medical expenses exceeding 10 percent of family income in 1980.

The high health care costs incurred by some children are associated with a variety of conditions and indicated medical treatments, including respiratory support and intravenous therapy. Such children may also require extensive nursing care. Between 1960 and 1984, the rate of chronic conditions among children under age 17 nearly tripled, rising from 1.8 percent (1.1 million children) to more than 5 percent (3.1 million children). At least part of the increase in chronic conditions among children reflects the success of health care providers in saving and maintaining the lives of congenitally or otherwise severely ill or impaired children. The health care costs of these children totaled nearly $4 billion in 1986 (Newacheck, 1987). The Office of Technology Assessment (OTA) estimates that between 2,300 and 17,000 children have conditions that require either respiratory support or intravenous therapy, together with continual and complex nursing attention. An additional 40,000 to 75,000 children may be dependent on less continual but still costly interventions to sustain life (U.S. Congress, 1987b).

Some catastrophic costs for children, particularly low birth weight newborns, may be preventable with appropriate prenatal care. Costs of intensive care services for newborns were estimated to be about $2.4 billion to $3.3 billion in 1985, averaging nearly $15,000 per case (U.S. Congress, 1987a). Estimates of how catastrophic neonatal costs might be reduced by improved prenatal care vary. One analysis concluded that providing prenatal care to women at risk of low-birth-weight infants would save more than $3 in costs for every $1 spent on prenatal care (Institute of Medicine, 1985).

As a strategy for avoiding costly neonatal intensive care, the Kennedy-Weicker minimum health care plan would mandate that employer plans cover prenatal care. Sen. John Chafee (R-RI) has introduced legislation (S.1537) to provide coverage under Title V of the Social Security Act for children who incur health care costs in excess of $50,000.

The growing population of AIDS victims is also likely to generate catastrophic health care expenses, particularly for those without health insurance. The number of people with AIDS is projected to increase 550 percent between 1986 and 1991, from 31,000 to nearly 173,000.

Victims of ARC (those with various chronic conditions of increasing severity among people infected by the AIDS virus, but not meeting the technical criteria for an AIDS diagnosis) are not included in official projections of costs. Recently, the Centers for Disease Control (CDC), the federal agency that monitors infectious diseases, expanded the definition of AIDS to include two conditions that were previously considered to associated with ARC: dementia and chronic wasting syndrome. This definitional change raises the number of recognized AIDS victims by 10 to 15 percent.

Persons diagnosed with AIDS are automatically eligible for Social Security disability payments, and become eligible for Medicare coverage 24 months after disability payments begin. Because typical survival time for AIDS victims ranges between 7 and 18 months, few AIDS victims are likely to qualify for Medicare coverage. However, as improvements in treatment prolong the lifespan of AIDS victims, more may become eligible for Medicare as well as the continued coverage from employer plans required by the Consolidated Omnibus Budget Reconciliation Act of 1985 (COBRA). People with AIDS related disabilities who meet income standards for Supplemental Security Income cash assistance are immediately eligible for Medicaid benefits to finance needed medical care.

Estimates of different payers' cost share for AIDS victims vary widely. Available data indicate that from 13 to 65 percent of AIDS victims are privately insured (Sisk, 1987). Medicaid is also estimated to have paid for the care of between 7 and 65 percent of AIDS patients. Projections of AIDS spending also vary. Spending on medical care alone for AIDS is projected to grow to between $4.0 billion and $10.7 billion in 1991 (Scitovsky and Rice, 1987). In another estimate (Pascal, 1987), cumulative medical costs for AIDS between 1986 and 1991 were predicted to range from $15.4 billion to $112.5 billion, with an intermediate estimate of $37.6 billion.

Because scientific understanding of AIDS is changing rapidly, estimating future costs from limited historical data is difficult. Eventual changes in the populations at risk might affect the size of the AIDS population and the costs of care for different payers. Since approximately 90 percent of AIDS victims are of working age, employer-sponsored health insurance plans could sustain substantially higher costs as the AIDS population increases.

Proposals to change the financing of care of AIDS victims are emerging. S.24, sponsored by Sen. Daniel Moynihan (D-NY), and its companion bill, H.R.276, sponsored by Rep. Ted Weiss (D-CT), would eliminate the current 24-month waiting period to receive Medicare coverage among people with the CDC definition of AIDS who qualify for Social Security disability payments.

Conclusion

Although data are available to estimate the prevalence of catastrophic health expenditures among the population, little is known about the major sources of costs for individuals or the effect of catastrophic costs on families' economic well-being. The relative importance of insurance coverage in protecting against catastrophic expenses depends on how catastrophic expenses are defined. If catastrophic expenses are defined as an absolute threshold amount of uninsured expenses, people with individual private insurance plans are most at risk. If catastrophic expenses are defined as uninsured expenditures exceeding some percentage of family income, the uninsured and the poor are at greatest risk. Participant cost sharing and limits on covered services can leave both publicly and privately insured persons at risk for catastrophic expenditures.

Pending legislative proposals attempt to address different issues related to catastrophic health care costs among the nonelderly population. One proposal (H.R. 2300) would guarantee minimum benefits in existing employer plans. Another (S. 1265) would require that employers provide most workers with health insurance that would include coverage of catastrophic health care costs. However, increasing the proportion of catastrophic costs that are insured by employer plans may increase premium costs for participants, or reduce basic coverage in employer plans. Although some families may benefit from improved catastrophic coverage, even with higher premiums and reduced basic coverage, most families may actually pay more out-of-pocket expenses to gain catastrophic protection. This tradeoff may make it difficult to enact legislation attempting to improve employer coverage for catastrophic health care costs in existing plans.

References

American Academy of Pediatrics, "Health Care Financing for the Child With Catastrophic Costs." June 1987. (Mimeographed.)

Chollet, Deborah, J. "Financing Indigent Health Care." In Frank B. McArdle, ed. *The Changing Health Care Market.* Washington, DC: Employee Benefit Research Institute, 1987.

Employee Benefit Research Institute. "A Profile of the Nonelderly Population without Health Insurance." *EBRI Issue Brief* 66 (May 1987).

_____. "AIDS: Potentially Costly to Employers and Employees." *Employee Benefit Notes* 5 (May 1987).

_____. "Features of Employer Health Plans: Cost Containment, Plan Funding, and Coverage Continuation." *EBRI Issue Brief* 60 (November 1986).

Farley, Pamela J. "Who Are the Underinsured?" *Health and Society* 3 (1985):476–503.

Institute of Medicine. National Academy of Sciences. *Preventing Low Birth Weight*. Washington, DC: National Academy Press, 1985.

InterStudy. *The InterStudy Edge: Quarterly Report of HMO Growth & Enrollment as of March 31, 1987*. (Summer 1987).

Newacheck, Paul. "The Cost of Caring for Chronically Ill Children." *Business and Health* 3 (January 1987).

Pascal, Anthony. *The Costs of Treating AIDS Under Medicaid*. Santa Monica, CA: The Rand Corporation, May 1987.

Scandlen, Gregory. "The Changing Environment of Mandated Benefits." *Employee Benefit Notes* 6 (June 1987):16.

Scitovsky, Anne A., and Dorothy P. Rice. "Estimates of the Direct and Indirect Costs of Acquired Immunodeficiency Syndrome in the United States, 1985, 1986, and 1991." *Public Health Reports* 102 (January-February 1987):5–17.

Sisk, Jane E. "The Cost of AIDS: A Review of the Estimates." *Health Affairs* 2 (Summer 1987):5–21.

U.S. Congress. House. Joint Hearing, Select Committee on Aging and Select Committee on Children, Youth, and Families. *Catastrophic Health Insurance: The Needs of Children*. 100th Cong., 1st. session, March 23, 1987. Washington, DC: U.S. Goverement Printing Office, 1987a.

U.S. Congress. Office of Technology Assessment. *Technology Dependent Children: Hospital v. Home Care*. Washington, DC: U.S. Government Printing Office, May 1987b.

U.S. Department of Labor. Bureau of Labor Statistics. *Employee Benefits in Medium and Large Firms, 1986*. Washington, DC: U.S. Government Printing Office, June 1987.

Wyszewianski, Leon. "Financially Catastrophic and High-Cost Cases: Definitions, Distinctions, and Their Implications for Policy Formulation." *Inquiry* 23 (Winter 1986):382–394.

V. A Social Insurance Approach to Long-Term Care

PAPER BY JOHN ROTHER, MARY JO GIBSON, AND THERESA VARNER

In June 1988 the 100th Congress enacted legislation to protect Medicare beneficiaries against catastrophic health care costs. Known as the Medicare Catastrophic Coverage Act of 1988, the legislation focuses largely on costs associated with acute medical episodes, and therefore fails to tackle the primary source of catastrophic costs for older Americans—long-term care.

If we are to provide Medicare beneficiaries with meaningful catastrophic protections, we must deal aggressively—and soon—with the issue of long-term care. To do so effectively, we must free the debate on long-term care from the narrow and constraining context of catastrophic illness.

Definitional Issues

Catastrophic illness has, of course, been defined variously but almost always in terms of cost. The following are the three most common definitions:

- Flat dollar expenditures for medical care, either incurred or out-of-pocket.

- Particular diseases or conditions we know to be associated with high costs.

- Expenditures expressed as a percentage of income, or "thresholds," reflecting "different degrees of sacrifice or financial consequences ... (Trapnell, Mays, and Tallis, 1983).

Both Wyszewianski (1986) and Berki (1986) note that financial ruin can accompany even modest medical expenditures when health coverage is absent or inadequate, and when income and other resources are insufficient to cover medical costs without producing undue harm. Indeed, Berki notes that in 1977, 80 percent of those families who spent more than 10 percent of their income on health care actually spent less than $2,000 in the course of the year.

Congress has not explicitly addressed the complex and thorny definitional issues whose resolution would seem to be critical to the rational development of public policy on catastrophic illness. But the design of the Medicare Catastrophic Coverage Act of 1988 *implicitly* reflects certain basic assumptions about the nature of the catastrophic medical experience among older Americans.

One underlying assumption seems to be that Medicare beneficiaries are indeed exposed to catastrophic risks from acute medical costs. The range and number of acute care benefits contained in the proposed legislation suggest a second implicit assumption, i.e., that the nature of the acute care experience for older Americans is a cumulative one. Finally, a third assumption appears to be that there is sufficient risk from acute care costs to justify a relatively radical departure from Medicare's existing financing mechanism to pay for expanded benefits. For the first time in the history of the Medicare program, beneficiaries alone would be expected to pay for the full cost of expanded benefits, and, for the first time, payments for such benefits would be linked to income.

The legislation does not provide complete protection against acute care costs, and the omissions are significant. For example, the legislation does not adequately address the formidable—and growing—burden of Medicare Part B costs on older Americans. In 1986, Medicare beneficiaries spent close to $3 billion out-of-pocket on "balance billing" by physicians unwilling to accept Medicare assignment. And the rise in the Part B premium for 1988 to $24.80 per month (up by more than 38 percent over 1987), and to about $30.90 in 1989, is particularly disturbing, for these increases suggest that current controls on Part B costs have not been entirely effective.

Long-Term Care as a Catastrophic Cost

Still, the single greatest source of catastrophic costs for older Americans is long-term care. Since the current congressional catastrophic insurance legislation does not deal in any meaningful way with the long-term care burden, the "catastrophic" label that has been so loosely applied is a misnomer.

Nursing home stays account for more than 80 percent of the expenses incurred by older persons who experience very high out-of-pocket costs for health care, i.e., over $2,000 per year (Rice and Gabel, 1986). Recent estimates of the economic burden of Alzheimer's disease to the patient and his or her family are even more staggering. According to Hay and Ernst, direct net costs (excluding such indirect costs as unpaid family care and lost productivity) amount to $9,600 per patient in the first year after diagnosis, and $8,700 per year thereafter (Hay and Ernst, 1987).

The need for long-term care leads almost inevitably to an unmanageable financial burden because the costs of care—whether delivered in an institution or at home—are often enormous. The cost of care in a nursing home now averages nationally over $22,000 per year, and the cost of home care can range from $50 to $200 per day.

As impressive as are the foregoing estimates of long-term care costs, their magnitude should not be permitted to obscure matters of equal weight in the development of long-term care policy. It is not at all clear that older Americans and society as a whole are well-served by framing the debate on long-term care issues in terms of the "catastrophic" experience. By adopting such a narrow "cost" focus, we may subordinate—or neglect entirely—equally important issues: the design of an effective delivery system of long-term care services, the right to autonomy and dignity in the use of those services, the quality of care provided, and support for family members in their role as caregivers.

This paper is intended to broaden the perspective from which we view the development of a national policy on long-term care. It undertakes to lay out the framework for a comprehensive long-term care social insurance program and to document the political feasibility of such an approach.

Why Private Long-Term Insurance Is Not the Answer

Over the past several years, much of the debate about long-term care financing has centered on the potential of private long-term care financing for solving the problem. The report by the Task Force on Long-Term Health Policies (U.S. Department of Health and Human Services, 1987), for example, focused solely on private-sector options, and offered a host of recommendations aimed at promoting private long-term care insurance. Yet the hope that such insurance will be able to reduce dramatically the burden of long-term care expenses on American families is likely to prove illusory.

The private long-term care insurance market confronts major problems in demand as well as supply. On the demand side, barriers include the cost of policies and the limits and restrictions in coverage. Also, many persons deny they will ever need such protection. The cost of policies that are available range from about $20 per month at age 55 to about $125 per month at age 75. Due to competing demands on their resources, many younger as well as older persons feel they cannot afford the premiums. Because indemnity plans are not adjusted for inflation, the protection they will offer in future years may be seriously eroded. In addition, most plans require a prior hospitalization and provide few, if any, benefits for home care. While some of the limitations may be remedied in future policies, better coverage and affordability will remain trade-offs (Wiener et al., 1987).

There are also serious problems on the supply side. Although the number of policies in force is said to have doubled from 1986 to 1987 (HHS, 1987), the market remains in its infancy. Although many insurers are "interested" in the market, few are sufficiently comfortable with their ability to price their policies to move aggressively. Most companies are going very slowly, establishing market "presence," but avoiding significant market penetration.

Tripling the number of persons covered by private long-term care insurance in the next few years would be a significant feat. Even if this were to be accomplished, however, only a very small fraction of the 51 million Americans age 55 and over, who are most likely to need such protection, would have coverage.

Projections by the Brookings Institution indicate that, even with very generous assumptions about who would participate, the proportion of total nursing home expenditures financed through private long-term care insurance by the years 2016–2020 will be in the very modest range of 7 to 12 percent (Rivlin and Wiener, 1988). The accompanying reductions in Medicaid expenditures are projected to be even smaller. The primary reasons for this small impact are that private-sector options have serious limitations and restrictions in coverage which reduce the protection they can offer, and most older persons cannot afford the costs. In summary, the evidence suggests that private long-term care insurance will not be a panacea to the long-term care financing problem and, at best, will become only a modest component of a much broader financing plan.

The Need for a Social Insurance Approach to Long-Term Care

It is sometimes argued that long-term care should be the responsibility of the private sector, not the government. This argument ignores the fact that our nation has had a long and successful tradition of providing protection through social insurance against risks that threaten the basic security of Americans. Social Security, for example, has proved effective in providing basic protection against the risk of lost earnings due to retirement, disability, and death. Medicare has made major strides in protecting acutely ill older people from unmanageable health care expenses. And Medicare is able to return about $.97 in benefits for every $1 of financing, a loss ratio which private insurance could never hope to achieve.

The very nature of long-term care also lends itself to a social insurance approach based on shared risk: (1) relatively few persons in our society need long-term care at any one time; (2) it is nearly impossible to predict who these individuals will be; and (3) the lifetime risk of needing nursing home care is much higher than most people think. Recent estimates of the lifetime risk of institutionalization at age 65, for example, range from 36 percent (Liang and Jow-Ching Tu, 1986) to 63 percent (McConnel, 1986).

These facts—along with the need to ensure access by all of those who may someday need long-term care—argue inherently for universal protection based on a social insurance approach to the problem. The costs to any one person will be small, while offering protection to all against catastrophic expenses. If spread across people's working lives, comprehensive long-term care coverage is certainly affordable. Moreover, these funds for insurance would come from shifting the burden away from the few who must now bear the brunt of the load to a broader population.

The Political Feasibility of a Social Insurance Approach

Long-term care reform has been called a "Rubic's cube," a complex maze, and a problem that defies solution. Widespread fears about the cost and complexity of reforming our nation's flawed long-term care system have contributed to an atmosphere in Washington policy circles of, at best, tentative incrementalism and, at worst, paralysis.

What seems to have been forgotten in the debate is that solutions to the problem, and even our vision of what is possible, directly interact with the general public's willingness to pay for services they perceive as essential to their well-being and security. A recent public opinion survey conducted by the American Association of Retired Persons (AARP) and the Villers Foundation sought to gauge support for long-term care reform among 1,000 registered voters of all ages (R.L. Associates, 1987). In brief, it was found that long-term care is an issue of nearly universal concern and high saliency, and Americans not only want an expanded federal program of long-term care but are willing to pay for it through increased taxes.

Among the poll's highlights:

- More than 60 percent of respondents have had direct experience with the need for long-term care. Almost half (47 percent) said that they or a family member, typically a spouse, parent, or grandparent, had needed long-term care; an additional 14 percent have close friends whose relatives have required such care. Among those without direct personal experience, more than half anticipate that it is very or fairly likely that someone in their family will need long-term care within the next five years.

- Over half of the respondents knew that Medicare rarely covers nursing home costs: 40 percent said Medicare pays for "only a little" nursing home care and 11 percent said "none."

- An overwhelming 86 percent of respondents, when asked to choose between "leaving long-term care entirely to the individual" and "it is time to consider some kind of government action," opted to involve the government.

- The great majority (84 percent) of those polled said it would be better if a government program of long-term care covered people of any age who are disabled, including children, rather than elderly people only.

- The majority (60 percent) agreed with the statement that "A government program of long-term care should be available to everyone, regardless of how rich or poor they are," rather than "long-term care is too expensive for the government to pay for everyone and should be a program only for poor people" (27 percent).

- The vast majority want a program that will provide home care as well as nursing home care. Support for home care is so strong that 65 percent of respondents said they still wanted home care even if "overall program costs would be much higher because more people would participate."

Perhaps most significantly, when asked if they personally would be willing to pay substantially increased monthly taxes to fund a federal program of long-term care for the elderly, the great majority (73 percent) of respondents—in all income groups—said yes (table V.1). It is notable that a majority (60 percent) even supported the highest cost program about which they were queried.

In summary, the poll results indicate that the lack of an adequate long-term care system is becoming a national family crisis and that support for change spans all age and income groups.

A Proposal for a Long-Term Care Social Insurance Program

It is not only the preoccupation with long-term care costs and financing that has impeded movement toward significant reform. Equally problematic has been the complexity of trying to redesign our fragmented service delivery system. Among the challenges are

TABLE V.1
Support for Long-Term Care Program for Persons 65 and Older, by Monthly Cost[a] (all income groups combined)

	Lowest Cost[b]	Middle Cost[c]	Highest Cost[d]
Number	334	332	330
Yes	73%	69%	60%
No	19	21	25
Don't know	8	9	12

[a]For each cost level, the monthly charge about which respondents were queried represented a fixed percentage of their income.
[b]Lowest cost for persons with incomes under $20,000 was $10 per month; for those with incomes from $20,000–$30,000, $15; and for those with incomes over $30,000, $25.
[c]Middle cost for persons with incomes under $20,000 was $15 per month; for those with incomes from $20,000–$30,000, $25; and for those with incomes over $30,000, $40.
[d]Highest cost for persons with incomes under $20,000 was $25 per month; for those with incomes from $20,000–$30,000, $40; and for those with incomes over $30,000, $60.

how to achieve a better integration of health and social services and of acute care and chronic care; improve the quality of both community-based and institutional services; maximize individual choice while controlling inappropriate utilization; encourage but not abuse the support families provide to frail older relatives; and respond effectively to the heterogenous needs of the many different groups who require long-term care.

There are no easy answers to these challenges. Yet, after well over a decade of experimentation with and research on long-term care reform, AARP, the Villers Foundation, and the Older Women's League (OWL) recently decided that the time had come to marshall existing knowledge and move forward with a comprehensive plan.

In the spring of 1987 these three organizations set in motion a process—not yet complete—to develop a long-term care social insurance proposal designed to protect a substantial portion of the population from the risks associated with the need for long-term care. This process entailed analyzing published long-term care reform proposals and convening an advisory committee of nationally recognized experts in the field of long-term care and disability.[1]

---

[1]The advisory committee members were: Robert Ball, Robert N. Butler, Carroll L. Estes, Judith Feder, Catherine Hawes, Robert L. Kane, Douglas Martin, Judy Meltzer, Anne R. Somers, and Joshua Wiener. Jack Needleman, Barbara Maynard, and Lynn Blewett of Lewin & Associates served as consultants to this process.

The proposed program, to be built on an expansion of Medicare, would provide a broad range of community-based and institutional care services to persons who are severely disabled. An innovative, two-tiered financing approach would establish separate financing mechanisms for future cohorts of retirees and for those who are currently retired or near retirement. Although beneficiary cost sharing would be required through copayments for both community and institutional care, persons with low incomes would be protected through an enhanced Medicaid program. The proposed administrative/service delivery system would be built around the concept of care coordination.

Outlined below are some of the key components of the proposal.

Insured Populations—The goal of the program is universal long-term care insurance coverage for persons of all ages with severe disabilities. Whether accomplished through immediate coverage or a phased approach, continued movement toward universal coverage for all of those in need of long-term care is a central tenet of the proposal.

The groups to be immediately covered would include all persons who currently qualify for Medicare acute care, including persons 65 and older and those who qualify for Medicare under Old-Age, Survivors and Disability Insurance (OASDI), including disabled workers, widows, widowers, and adult disabled children of covered workers.

One of the problematic aspects of linking coverage decisions to OASDI eligibility is that OASDI is based on a philosophy of wage replacement and hence does not cover children and adults who have never been able to work due to their disability but who nonetheless need long-term care. The sponsoring organizations and the advisory committee members have been struggling to find ways to provide meaningful benefits, consistent with proposed financing, to those disabled groups *not* covered under OASDI/Medicare. These groups consist of children under 18, including disabled children of covered workers and disabled adults judged able to engage in "substantial gainful employment."

A major barrier to decisionmaking about the inclusion of groups not currently covered under OASDI/Medicare has been the lack of any reliable published estimates of the cost of providing long-term care services to persons under age 65. AARP has recently contracted with ICF, Incorporated to model these costs. One of the options under discussion would be to phase in coverage, in the very near future, of community-based services for children and adults not covered under OASDI. The exact timing of the phase-in and the specific services that might be covered have not yet been determined, pending cost estimates.

Service Eligibility—The program would provide services to persons who are severely physically or mentally disabled. "Severe disability" is defined conceptually as the need for a level of care comparable to that provided in an intermediate care facility (ICF), although one need not be institutionalized to receive services. Because the definitional issues are complex, the secretary of the Department of Health and Human Services would be asked to establish a new commission to refine the criteria for level of need/benefit determinations, taking into account the need for help with activities of daily living (ADLs). While it is necessary to specify a minimum number of ADL dependencies, such as three, in order to model cost estimates, this is insufficient in and of itself for determining who should qualify for services. The commission would also take into account the need for supervision/behavior monitoring and the need for skilled nursing care.

Covered Services—The proposed program would pay for a broad range of community and institutional services, including skilled nursing facility (SNF) and ICF care, skilled nursing at home, case management, home health care, personal care, adult day care, respite care, mental health counseling, functional assessment and care planning, habilitation, and rehabilitation services to maintain functioning. The services listed are intended to be representative of client needs.

Utilization would be controlled by providing a defined set of services to each beneficiary, with the assessment/screening function to be conducted by community-based "care coordination" organizations. (See discussion of the administrative mechanisms below.) Utilization would also be controlled through beneficiary copayments.

Copayments and Deductibles—There would be no front-end deductible for either institutional or community services. The rationale for this decision was that there is little empirical evidence that deductibles help control inappropriate utilization among persons age 65 and over. Instead, they serve as a barrier to access to needed care.

Flat (non-income-related) copayments would begin on the first day a beneficiary used either institutional or community services. However, so that current benefits under Medicare's postacute program are not reduced, the copayments would begin only when a person no longer qualified for Part A coverage.

The proposed copayment rates are set at 30 percent of charges for nursing home care and 20 percent for community-based care. The rationale for these levels is that the program should not pay for "room and board" costs of nursing home care; and there should be no financial incentive to use one part of the system (i.e., community or institutional care) over another.

Low Income Protection—Those with low income would be protected by an expanded Medicaid program designed to pick up the copayments for persons with incomes at or below 150 percent (or possibly 200 percent) of the federal poverty line. There would also be additional protections to prevent the impoverishment of spouses of nursing home residents and an increased "personal needs allowance" for residents. The savings achieved by the current Medicaid program as a result of the new social insurance program could be used to help finance these additional protections for low-income individuals.

Financing—The proposed financing approach reflects the need to rely on traditional sources of financing for social insurance programs. It also reflects the desire to spread costs equitably across the general population on an income-related basis and between the retired and working-age population.

An innovative, two-tiered financing scheme, first conceptualized by Marilyn Moon (Moon, 1986), would establish separate financing mechanisms for future cohorts of retirees and for those who are currently retired or near retirement.

For working-age Americans, benefits could be financed through increased payroll taxes. This financing method would allow very substantial reserves to accumulate and would likely provide for fully funded benefits by the time the earliest cohorts of the "baby boom" generation reach retirement age.

Transitional financing monies would be required to "grandfather" in persons who are currently retired or near retirement and hence unable to make substantial prior contributions to the program via the payroll tax. A combination of dedicated taxes could be used as transitional monies, including an income tax surcharge, higher estate taxes, and "sin" taxes on cigarettes and alcohol. Any income tax surcharge and possibly estate and "sin" taxes could be phased out over time as reserves accumulate.

Finally, general revenues could be used to help subsidize a means-tested program similar to Medicaid to provide protection for persons with low incomes.

Administrative Mechanisms—In proposing various administrative mechanisms, we recognize that our society has not yet found the "best" methods of delivering long-term care services. Hence the structure of the system needs to foster continued innovation and a flexible response to client needs.

We also recognize that, in the traditional spirit of American individualism, most citizens would prefer to have practically unlimited choice in determining what services they need and who will provide them. In our nation's acute care system, patients and their physicians are usually the sole "gatekeepers" to services. Yet, from a health policy viewpoint, we know that we need to control utilization and cost of long-term care services by using "care coordinators" to channel clients to the most cost-effective forms of care. We also know that care coordinators can help direct clients to the mix of services which is most appropriate to their needs. Thus, the challenge is to build a system of care coordination that respects individual preferences and autonomy while it also protects the public purse.

We are currently discussing the possibility of allowing beneficiaries to opt for either of two different plans. The first model, which we call "contractual coordinated care," is based on the traditional fee-for-service system. In this model, the federal government would contract with care coordination agencies, such as area agencies on aging or state agencies, to conduct level of care/benefit determinations, develop care plans, coordinate services, and monitor the quality of care provided. These organizations, in turn, would contract with local providers, who would be paid on a fee-for-service basis, to deliver services.

In the second model, which we call "modified capitation," the federal government would contract with community-based care coordination agencies and pay them on a capitated basis. Beneficiaries would be able to choose and switch plans during open season. The agencies would be required to assume risk, be not-for-profit or state/county owned, perform all needed functions, and have strong consumer and community representation on their boards. These agencies would be monitored by the federal government, possibly through contracts with the states.

Clearly, it will be critical to have strong quality assurance mechanisms in these managed care systems. (Our proposals for quality assurance, as well as for provider reimbursement, are beyond the scope of this paper.)

Why the Proposal Will Not Lead to Runaway Costs

Concerns are often expressed that the "floodgates" of demand will be opened and that families will shift their responsibilities to formal providers if public benefits for long-term care are expanded. Yet research in the United States and many other industrialized nations indicates that this will not be the case. Community-based long-term care services have been offered in a number of other countries for some time without runaway utilization. In Manitoba, Canada, for example, comprehensive home care services have been available since 1975 to all residents at no out-of-pocket cost and based solely on professionally assessed need. Between 1975 and 1978, roughly 10 percent of persons aged 65 and over (Shapiro, 1986) received home care services at some point each year, with this figure dropping to 7 percent between 1985 and 1986 (Fletcher, 1987).

A wide body of research in the United States also indicates that families do not significantly reduce the amount of assistance they are providing when formal services are introduced (Mathematica Policy Research, 1986) and that older persons and their family caregivers tend to underutilize those services that are available in relation to objective need (Hawes et al., 1987).

The Canadian experience also offers reassurance in this respect. Although most long-term care services are available to Canadian citizens at relatively little out-of-pocket cost, family support remains strong, and there is little evidence of inappropriate institutionalization. Moreover, the percentage of gross national product (GNP) devoted to health care in Canada, which includes many long-term care services under its universal health care system, is significantly less than in the United States—8.6 percent in Canada in 1985 compared with 10.7 percent in the United States.

The Time Is Now

The proposal outlined above is far from perfect and needs considerable refinement. Nonetheless, we do believe that we have the contours of a workable and equitable plan, and we know that we are way ahead of where we were just a few years ago.

Policymakers cannot afford to delay much longer in alleviating the catastrophic financial burdens experienced by Americans who need long-term care. Younger as well as older citizens are growing impatient with the lack of movement toward meaningful long-term care reform. Many older Americans live in fear that they will be a burden on their children or be forced to relinquish their life savings to afford care in a nursing home. Many adult children fear that they will not be able to give their parents the help that they may need. Our poll data suggest that long-term care is an issue of great emotional depth, and it is one that we believe will soon translate into political action.

In our recent poll, surprisingly high percentages of voters said they would be more likely to vote for a presidential candidate who supported a federal program of long-term care, and less likely to vote for a candidate who opposed such a program. In addition, almost three-quarters (73 percent) of respondents said that a candidate who would support a program of long-term care "shows the kind of leadership and vision I would like."

What once was perceived as a purely personal problem is now being perceived as one for society as a whole. During the last 50 years, the avoidance of economic catastrophe for the aging family has been translated into major action twice—in 1935, through the enactment of Social Security, and in 1965, through the enactment of Medicare. Brody (1987) has argued that the ruinous cost of long-term care is the third such catastrophe for aging families and that the perception of the problem in economic terms is the catalyst for policy change. We believe that this perception is rapidly growing and becoming, in Brody's words, a new "felt necessity of the times."

References

Berki, S.E. "A Look at Catastrophic Medical Expenses and the Poor." *Health Affairs* 5 (Winter 1986): 138–144.

Brody, Stanley J. "Strategic Planning: The Catastrophic Approach." *The Gerontologist* 27 (1987): 132.

Fletcher, Susan. "Cost and Financing of Long-Term Care in Canada." In Mary Jo Gibson, ed. *Income Security and Long-Term Care for Women in Midlife and Beyond: U.S. and Canadian Perspectives.* Washington, DC: American Association of Retired Persons, 1987.

Hay, Joel W., and Richard L. Ernst. "The Economic Costs of Alzheimer's Disease." *American Journal of Public Health* 77 (September 1987): 9.

Hawes, Catherine; Rosalie Kane; Linda L. Powers; and James Reinardy. "Lessons About Home and Community-Based Long-Term Care." Paper. Washington, DC: American Association of Retired Persons, 1988.

Liang, Jersey, and Edward Jow-Ching Tu. "Estimating Lifetime Risk of Nursing Home Residency: A Further Note." *The Gerontologist* 26 (1986).

Mathematica Policy Research, Inc. *The Evaluation of the National Long-Term Demonstration: Analysis of the Benefits and Costs of Channeling.* Prepared for U.S. Department of Health and Human Services. Washington, DC: U.S. Government Printing Office, 1986.

McConnel, Charles E. "A Note on the Lifetime Risk of Nursing Home Residence." *The Gerontologist* 24 (December 1986).

Moon, Marilyn. "Changing the Structure of Medicare." Unpublished paper. Summer 1986.

Rice, Thomas, and Jon Gabel. "Protecting the Elderly Against High Health Care Costs." *Health Affairs* 3 (Fall 1986): 16.

Rivlin, Alice M., and Joshua M. Wiener. *Caring for the Disabled Elderly: Who Will Pay?* Washington, DC: The Brookings Institution, 1988.

R.L. Associates. *The American Public Views Long Term Care: A Survey Conducted for the AARP and the Villers Foundation.* Princeton, NJ: R.L. Associates, 1987.

Shapiro, Evelyn. "Patterns and Predictors of Home Care by the Elderly When Need Is the Sole Basis for Admission." *Home Health Services Quarterly* 7 (Spring 1986): 38.

Trapnell, Gordon R.; James W. Mays; and Inger M. Tallis. *Strategies for Insuring Catastrophic Illness: Financial Burden, Prototype Plans, and Cost Estimates.* Nutley, NJ: Hoffman-La Roche, Inc., 1983, p.88.

U.S. Department of Health and Human Services. *Report to Congress and the Secretary by the Task Force on Long Term Health Care Policies.* Washington: DC, U.S. Government Printing Office, 1987.

Wiener, Joshua M.; Deborah Ehrenworth; and Denise A. Spence. "Private Long-Term Care Insurance: Cost, Coverage, and Restrictions." *The Gerontologist* 27 (August 1987): 493.

Wyszewianski, Leon. "Financially Catastrophic and High-Cost Cases: Definitions, Distinctions, and Their Implications for Policy Formulation." *Inquiry* 23 (Winter 1986): 382–384.

VI. Part Two Discussion

MR. ROTHER: I have about ten observations that I hope will be provocative and build on what has already been said today.

First, it is an error to look at health policy solely in terms of catastrophic coverage. The only reason we are here today talking about the issue of catastrophic insurance is that one individual, Dr. Otis Bowen, decided to take up a very old idea, namely, a stop-loss concept under Medicare and push it through as his legacy as Secretary of HHS. That is the only reason we are using *catastrophic* as a guide in health policy.

I do not think the primary actors in health policy today would have defined catastrophic as the principal policy goal with regard to either the older or the younger population today. The basic goals are access, quality, and cost. Those have always been the goals. And catastrophic, in many ways, blinds us to those goals because it defines and frames the issues solely in terms of financial protection.

Let me address Leon Wyszewianski's point about ability to pay versus the stop-loss concept. The fundamental public policy basis of Medicare has always been simply to continue for the aged and disabled population the basic mainstream insurance arrangements that most enjoyed while employed. And it was no accident that Medicare simply tried to replicate the standard Blue Cross-Blue Shield policy in effect in 1965. In that sense, the current effort in Congress to put in stop-loss features in Medicare is really an old policy because we are simply trying to make Medicare's coverage conform to prevailing private insurance arrangements.

Balance Billing and Long-Term Care

I think that explains why catastrophic legislation is so overwhelmingly popular and why, in some respects, it is really not any major advancement but rather simply a catch-up. When we talk about some other areas, however, then we are talking about some truly new areas that may push Medicare beyond most private health insurance arrangements. This certainly involves long-term care, but also involves the problem of balance billing by physicians, which is still a catastrophic risk faced by many older persons today.* And, paradoxically,

---

*Editor's note: Balance billing is billing for the balance of charges that are not reimbursed by Medicare.

73

even with the addition of a prescription drug benefit to Medicare, there is no stop-loss on that prescription provision.

Thus, speaking for the over-65 population, the principal risks in a financial sense remaining after enactment of catastrophic insurance legislation will be balance billing by physicians and long-term care.

Second, I should mention that about a third of American Association of Retired Persons' (AARP) membership is under the age of 65. A third of our members are working full time, and we have a very strong interest in various proposals to require stop-loss coverage in the private sector. We clearly have a major problem with health insurance coverage, particularly for those people in their 50s and early 60s who have conditions that may preclude any normal insurance coverage, for people who are working part time, and for displaced homemakers going back to work in service-sector jobs.

We are also concerned, however, about the mandated benefit approach, such as the one proposed by Sen. Edward Kennedy (D-MA)* because of the potential impact, depending on how it is structured, on job opportunities. This is particularly an issue for part-time older workers, who may see significant new employment barriers arise because of the costs of mandated benefits.

Nonetheless, the issue of the availability of coverage is a growing one for our members in terms of concerns about their children and their grandchildren. It does seem to me that Congress is likely to turn its attention eventually to the issue of catastrophic coverage for those under 65.

I would still argue that a strictly catastrophic approach is the wrong way to frame this issue, but it certainly seems to be the cheapest way to approach it. It will be an attractive way for Congress to continue to look at the health issue.

The Rising Costs of Compensation for Doctors

Third, let me go back to the problem of doctors and balance billing. This is not a problem confined to older people alone. Doctors determine health care costs and utilization in our society. How we, in our various insurance arrangements, decide to compensate doctors has probably a decisive impact on total health care expenditures.

Recent increases in Part B premiums of 38 percent in one year are a radicalizing event for both Congress and the public, and they will force Congress to deal directly with a program that is now out of

*Editor's note: Senator Kennedy's bill (S. 1265), the Minimum Health Benefits for All Workers Act.

control. It is a little early to predict exactly how this will happen, but I submit that rising physician costs are a problem not only for Medicare but also for just about every private insurance arrangement as well, because these increases are not confined simply to the population over 65.

The easiest way for older people to respond to this problem is to demand mandatory assignment. The Supreme Court has recently let stand the Massachusetts requirement that every doctor in the state, as a condition of licensure, accept assignment under the Medicare program. There are also several ballot initiatives, most prominently in the state of Washington, to require mandatory assignment. The Supreme Court decision may give a very substantial boost to those efforts. We know from our own polling that it is hard to find a more popular proposition among older people than a proposition that Medicare should be enough to pay 80 percent of the doctor bill, and they should not have to make more than the 20 percent statutory copayment.

I think there will be quite a bit of legislative activity in the area of physician fee reform. Medicare's policies ought to be coordinated with private sector policies because, if they are not, we are likely to see major dislocations and run the risk of a two-tier, second-class system under Medicare. There should be a very strong joint employer, insurer, and public interest in changing the way physicians are paid.

Long-Term Care: A Risk for the Family

Fourth, long-term care is clearly the principal focus of public debate when we talk about catastrophic issues in 1988 and beyond.

Increasingly long-term care is being seen not just as an individual risk but as a risk for the family. The point has already been made that the traditional picture we have of a well-defined family unit is increasingly less realistic now, with blended families and great geographical separation between parents and children. The whole idea of family responsibility is in serious need of shoring up through public policy.

Fifth, exclusive reliance on private-sector solutions, in effect, condemns the current generation of older persons to contend with the spend-down principle inherent in the current welfare approach to long-term care. It is simply not economically possible to ask people who are already so close to the time of highest risk to engage in risk spreading over a very short period of time. Premiums are too high to be affordable for most older persons.

75

In the summer of 1987, AARP, through the Prudential Insurance Company, made a private, individual long-term policy available for all of our members. We will continue to do that again on an open-period basis, but it is an age-related premium. Premiums are reasonable for those who get in early and young enough, but for those most at risk, namely, those in their 70s, the premiums go up to over $120 a month. So it should not surprise anyone that very, very few people have taken advantage of the offer.

As we meet a public demand for action, what we are going to see is what we have already seen in Medicare and Social Security, namely, a division of responsibility. The current generation of those at risk almost inevitably will need to be a public responsibility, whereas those now working and their dependents could easily be a private responsibility while they are in the active workforce, through an employer-based insurance arrangement.

Avoiding Spousal Impoverishment

Sixth, one interesting feature that did not gain much public attention in the catastrophic insurance legislation is the spousal impoverishment provision. Under Medicaid, the spouse remaining in the community is, in effect, forced on welfare for the rest of his or her life. The legislation allows the spouse remaining in the community to retain a certain amount of income and assets after the other spouse goes into a nursing home. This change is an early sign that Congress is ready to move away from a welfare approach to long-term care.

This is a fairly radical change in Medicaid policy. It basically reflects a recognition that a welfare-based policy in this area is a failure, and it reflects the surprising readiness of Congress to move toward more insurance-based approaches for long-term care. It is the first step, and significantly, it has been embraced by both conservatives and liberals, Republicans and Democrats. There is practically no opposition to this basic idea.

Service Delivery and Managed Care

Seventh, it is dangerous to define long-term care issues solely in terms of catastrophic care because that definition looks only at financial protection, not at service delivery and how the necessary care can best be managed.

The key element that must be built into long-term care is an infrastructure that is ready to manage this kind of service delivery. It is going to require a very heavy public investment to create that infrastructure, perhaps in conjunction with a private partnership.

We do not have places in our communities that we can turn to to manage long-term care services. In many communities, we don't even have referral or consulting services. Without a strong public investment in at least this much, we are going to have a very difficult problem managing what must be a very flexible benefit to be successful.

Along these lines, the impact of deficit-reduction could be devastating on the limited infrastructure we do have in community services, namely, Meals-on-Wheels, Senior Companions, and the Older Americans Act.

The Canadian System

Eighth, those of us who are serious about long-term care should look very carefully at Canada. Not that we can import a Canadian system wholesale, but there are a couple of things they do that we should consider. One is that the financing of long-term care is tied to the overall health-financing system, which means that they are able to shift funds from acute inpatient care to community-based services. It is very smart fiscal policy to tie those two together.

The Canadian system is also very flexible about defining benefits. There is a terrific ability at the local level to do whatever needs to be done to keep people functioning at home and out of an institution. I do not think the U.S. Congress is capable of writing a defined benefit design that preserves sufficient flexibility at the local level to keep people independent, which is actually Congress' goal. And I wonder how successfully we are going to do that in private-sector programs as well.

There needs to be a very strong case management infrastructure tied to comprehensive financing. And very flexible benefits.

When long-term benefits were begun in Canada, their use increased for about two years and then leveled off. There has been no extraordinary demand for the benefits because families prefer to continue to care for parents in the home. There has been no foisting off on public systems of family responsibilities.

Long-Term Care as a Problem for the Nonelderly

Ninth, we should not define long-term care primarily as a problem involving the elderly. Cost estimates show that the total annual cost of caring for those needing long-term care assistance in our society is about evenly divided between those over 65 and those under 65. There are a lot more people who need such care over the age of 65, but they need it for shorter periods of time. Those under 65 who need it, need it for a whole lifetime, and so the total cost is about evenly divided.

Even in political terms, the strongest constituency for long-term care action is not necessarily those over 65. The polling data show, in fact, that middle-aged people are most anxious, and this obviously reflects a combination of concern about their own as well as about their parents' futures. As the baby boom generation moves into the middle-aged years, we will see an explosion of interest in this issue. That will be reflected politically, as well, in demand for benefits in the private sector.

The definition of catastrophic is not, to me, the issue. The issue is, what the public wants and what the felt need of the times is politically. I would define this want as an insurance approach that deals with the issues of access, quality, and cost containment—an approach that strengthens families' ability to meet increasing demands on them. In my view, the public sector will be the focus for approaches that are targeted at those not in the labor force, namely, those who are retired or who are disabled, while the private sector will be the focus of policy efforts to support employers in meeting their responsibilities to their own current employees and their dependents.

A Market for Private Insurance?

MR. LANE: In the proposal by AARP, the Villers Foundation, and the Older Workers League, I was struck by the fact that there is 30 percent daily coinsurance for nursing home care and 20 percent coinsurance for home care. That, obviously, leaves a market for a private insurance vehicle very similar to a Medicare supplemental policy. Do you perceive this, then, as being an approach that would not preclude a realistic role for the private market in providing long-term care?

MR. ROTHER: I think that it would not preclude supplementary coverage at all. The basis for at least the institutional copayment is simply to reflect that we do have a retirement income system in this country that should be adequate for paying for room and board for most people. There is no need to have an insurance program that duplicates income that should already be available to cover it. It really reflects not so much a policy of saying: "Let's encourage people to go out and buy supplementary coverage" as it says: "We already have a Social Security system that should be adequate to handle this part of the bill. Let's not create a more expensive system than we need for that."

MR. LANE: It seems interesting, given Medicare and the discussion of Medicare supplemental insurance, that the growth of that market did, in fact, occur once the public sector commitment was well defined. Once that public sector was well defined, it created a significant niche for a market product. As I read the design, I immediately saw a major niche for a supplemental product to a public response. I wondered whether that was considered by the designer.

MR. ROTHER: It was considered. But our main goal is to keep the cost as reasonable as possible and yet have benefits that are adequate enough for everyone so it does not become simply an insurance program that is only of use to high-income people with substantial reserves and assets to supplement their benefits.

MS. FELICE: I think you could say there is no means-testing in the copayment you suggest in your comments on public subsidies for buy-in. Could you comment on your organization's philosophy on means testing?

MR. ROTHER: Anyone who knows AARP over its history knows that if there is one thing that characterizes our public policy positions, it is that we prefer insurance to welfare, and this is especially so for long-term care.

Means testing, in a strict sense, is a welfare approach, and that is why we have always had problems with it. The approach taken by Congress in Medicare catastrophic legislation is certainly not something we consider as means testing, but it reflects the need for taking into account differences in ability to pay when you set premiums. But, for a number of reasons, we would be strongly opposed to any differential benefits based on ability to pay, the principal reason being that such a policy would bring with it all the problems that we have experienced with welfare approaches. Other problems are more practical. For instance, as Laurence Lane mentioned, how can you possibly have a supplemental private benefit if you have a variable public benefit? So I think it is simply not a workable solution to try to take income into account on the benefit side.

MR. HICKOX: Do you foresee the possibility of federal legislative or regulatory action that would address balance billing or could such a thing occur only in a state as liberal as Massachusetts?

MR. ROTHER: I think two things are going to happen. The states are going to force the federal hand because some states are going to require doctors to accept assignment and other states will not. That will create popular pressure for uniformity.

Secondly, the 38 percent, one-year increase in Medicare premiums to both beneficiaries and to the federal Treasury is shaking up everyone who counseled moderation. The perception now is that we have to act and we have to act fast. What can we do? There is no easy answer to that but, certainly, most of the health leadership on Capitol Hill is committed to trying to take on the problem.

Serious cost cutting is a dangerous thing to address in Medicare alone. It is a problem that characterizes all health insurance. To prevent significant dislocations, we ought to work in such a way that whatever is done in the public sector is mirrored in the private sector or that there are parallel steps in the private sector.

A Two-Tiered Financing System

MS. MULLEN: Would you expand your comment on the possible role for the private sector in covering the working-age population? You talk about a two-tiered financing system in your paper and payroll taxes for coverage of the working-age population. How would that work?

MR. ROTHER: In the traditional social insurance system, you pay over the course of your working life to ensure that you have benefits when you are not working. This is a valid principle to apply to today's workers. If they pay small amounts out of each paycheck over a working life, then there should be a system in place that is adequately funded to take care of them when they retire.

What is tricky is handling the current generation of retirees who have not had the opportunity to pay in over a working life. You might want to consider a separate type of financing for that group that would be based more on dedicated general revenues such as estate taxes or a laundry list of other choices. The measures taken to finance the cost of the current generation would be temporary. Then it could honestly be said to people now working that the contributions they are being asked to make are for their future care.

MS. MULLEN: Then you are talking about a public-sector trust fund build up, such as Social Security, and not a private insurance program, which also relies on prefunding?

MR. ROTHER: There is a need for private-sector coverage in the first instance for people currently working and their dependents. This does not generally exist in our society. Until we deal with this problem, it seems premature to think about what the private-sector supplementary role ought to be for the already disabled or the 65-and-older population.

There is a primary responsibility that is still not being met in the private sector for those active employees and their dependents.

Is Supplemental Insurance Still Viable for Medicare Beneficiaries?

MR. VLADECK: There are 18 million Medigap policies out there. With a federal catastrophic insurance program, the people who write those policies are either going to have to reduce their premiums or find new benefits to sell. Is there a short-term strategic issue there in terms of movement toward better coverage of Medicare beneficiaries?

MR. ROTHER: I think that many in Congress hoped that the Medicare Catastrophic Coverage Act of 1988 would make it unnecessary for Medicare beneficiaries to have to buy supplementary policies, but the terms of the legislation are restrictive enough so that very few people are going to want to risk not having supplemental coverage.

Most retired people are understandably very risk averse and, indeed, do not want to run that kind of risk. So, I foresee a very small impact on consumer demand for supplemental coverage as a result of this legislation. In theory, the price should go down for supplemental coverage, but health cost increases have been on a steep slope. Most of the people I have talked to say that the new program will help, but there will still be increases—they just will not be as high as they would have otherwise been.

MR. SALISBURY: There is an interesting economic issue that arises with the supplemental insurance. The United Mine Workers (UMW) just did a survey of their retirees. The UMW provides a 100 percent fill-in against Medicare to all their worker retirees, yet they found that fully 30 percent of their current retirees are currently buying Medigap policies because they do not understand that they have protection. It would be interesting to determine what percentage of the Medigap market is made up of individuals who do not actually need the coverage.

81

MR. VLADECK: Can we use your point as a paradigm for all the discussion today about long-term care insurance?

Developing a Community-Based Long-Term Care System

MS. IGNAGNI: I am curious about John Rother's observations on the lack of a sophisticated infrastructure for a home health care delivery system. That probably explains why, thus far, the insurers have chosen to go the indemnity route based on institutional care. I think all of us agree that we need to do something else in developing a truly long-term community-based system.

Probably all of us would accept as a given that we are facing a bit of a challenge with respect to the Pepper bill, which contemplates a rather sophisticated infrastructure to achieve its objectives. If, indeed, we are on a fast track with respect to this type of legislation, how do you wrestle with that?

MR. ROTHER: It is a bit of a chicken-and-egg problem. Why should an infrastructure be created if there is no "insured population?" And yet, how can you create an insured population and be responsible to it without having a structure that is capable of managing what clearly requires careful management? The Pepper bill did not really solve that problem.

The only thing that seems responsible to me is a phased-in approach that simultaneously builds both an insured population and a structure to manage care. But it will not be easy. The really hard job in long-term care is to give those who are building the structure enough freedom to do it in the most cost-effective manner possible. I do not know right now that we have anyone to whom we can delegate that responsibility. There has to be as much or more emphasis on developing that infrastructure as on the terms of the actual insurance coverage.

MS. YOUNG: Right now we have people coming out of medical school with huge burdens of debt. Most of the material from the American Medical Association seems to indicate that by the time young doctors finish paying off debts and buying equipment, they are really in a fairly precarious financial position. Also, they are at an age when many of them are starting families. Yet we have an aging population. More of the people going into doctors' offices are going to be older, requiring more medical care, and expecting to be recipients of the blessings of American research. Under these circumstances, what will we do to our system if we respond through state and eventually federal programs that tell doctors they can no longer bill Medicare patients?

Has anybody tried to determine whether or not there is a level of profit that could be used to sustain the private system? What will we do to our system if the states follow through on the Supreme Court decision in the Massachusetts case?*

MR. ROTHER: Congress has been fairly crude about it in terms of imposing physician fee limitations.** The experience of the fee freeze was that physician net income during the freeze went up 16 percent in one year, and as soon as the freeze came off, a cost explosion occurred, even though there are still some limits in the Part B fees. So it has not been a very successful experience.

The problem is not simply one of freezing fees or even mandatory assignment. The problem is that the current system rewards the wrong kind of doctors and the wrong kinds of behavior of those doctors. It rewards invasive, aggressive medicine and penalizes doctors who take the time to talk to their patients and who are conservative in their approach. That is bad for Medicare; it is bad for our health system as a whole; and, in many cases, it is very bad for health outcomes. The right way to fix this is to shift the way we compensate doctors. We should reward those doctors who are doing the right things more than they are rewarded now. Once we get a fair payment system in place, we should make it pay-in-full so we also protect those who are supposed to be insured.

Priorities of Health Care

MR. LIFSON: I have a comment and also a question. The comment has to do with the payroll tax requirements of the proposed expanded benefit. As I understand it, the benefit would be fully funded at the point when individuals are in need of care. Such full funding assumes

---

*Editor's note: Over the last few years, four states—Massachusetts, Vermont, Rhode Island, and Connecticut—have enacted legislation that requires physicians to accept Medicare assignment. The Supreme Court recently refused to consider the appeal of a federal court decision upholding the Massachusetts statute (*Massachusetts Medical Society v. Dukakis*, 484 U.S. (1987), cert. denied). This precedent may lead to similar legislation in other states.
**Editor's note: The Deficit Reduction Act of 1984 (DEFRA) froze Medicare "customary, prevailing, and reasonable" (CPR) payments for one year.

that there would be large reserves set aside, which would produce extra public savings. At the same time we are faced with stock market uncertainty and budget deficits, which are staying the same or possibly going up.

One-third of the uninsured should be eligible for Medicaid. But the public sector—both the federal government and the states—keep saying: "We do not have the money to take care of the people who we said we were going to take care of."

I just wonder about the priorities of introducing yet another public benefit that will take funds into the public sector and probably end up costing more than anybody anticipates, by a significant factor.

MR. ROTHER: First, I will not quarrel with priorities. There are many priorities of health care, and I am speaking to only one of them. We are very concerned about those who lack any health coverage. Increasingly, our members feel a concern about their children and their grandchildren going without basics in preventive health, child immunization, and standard access to care.

Second, when we talk about long-term care, basically, we are talking about money that is being spent already. Some of it is not being spent very wisely, and almost all of it is being spent in a very unpredictable and unbudgetable fashion.

Our proposal, according to the models we have run, does not entail very much of an increase in total spending. It does entail a rearrangement in the financing of that spending on a more predictable basis.

MR. LIFSON: People said the total cost for Medicare would be rather modest and predictable, and it has proven to be anything but that.

MR. ROTHER: Which is why we will not create an open-ended cost-plus-reimbursement system. I think we have learned from our experience. Again, in Canada, a system has been developed in which access is provided and cost-containment features were built in from the start, apparently very successfully.

MR. MERRILL: John, is your preference for a public-sector long-term care program over a private-sector long-term care program premised on the fact that the private sector has been able to insure only 80 percent to 85 percent of the nonelderly?

MR. ROTHER: I was talking about long-term care. What I said was that a primary reliance on a private-sector strategy for long-term care would, I believe, have the effect of consigning almost all of the

84

present generation of older people to the welfare-based system that we have today. I do not think that is acceptable as a public policy response. We must have a policy that addresses current problems as well as the future needs of people who are currently working. I do not see a private-sector approach on the horizon that can deal with the current generation of retirees.

Employer Coverage of Long-Term Care for Retirees

MR. McCORMACK: Are the two employers who are developing a program for their employees going to pick up existing retirees under that program?

Ms. GAGLIARDI: We expect to offer it to retirees.

MR. McCORMACK: American Express will. What about John Hancock?

Ms. SCHAEFFER: We also will offer it to retirees, but only up to age 79.

MR. ROTHER: When Medicare was enacted in 1965, it was the national judgment that older people did not have access to health care financing. In fact, about one-third of that population had health insurance but two-thirds did not. If we ever managed to insure one-third of the current population, all of us would be rejoicing, but the public judgment would still be that that is not enough to solve the problem.

MR. McCORMACK: I do not think employers who are bringing this coverage to their employees are limiting it only to active employees. I think that should be made very clear. Any experience with these policies I have ever had, including the two that you have just heard about, do extend to current retirees. It is a big bridge to cross because it is an expensive one.

Ms. BORZI: John Rother is absolutely right. The reason long-term coverage is not going to be a feasible private-sector solution for the current retired population is that the cost is going to be prohibitive.

I am very happy to hear that American Express and John Hancock are going to offer long-term care coverage to their retirees, but I want to know what the cost is going to be for that 60-year-old, 65-year-old, 70-year-old person. In most instances, the mere cost is going to be a denial of access, not that the coverage is not freely available, but that people cannot afford it.

Ms. IGNAGNI: Although you can commend the corporations for taking some leadership on this issue, it would be irresponsible to suggest that the private sector is going to solve the problem. You are talking about a question of cost-shifting to the beneficiary or to the potential beneficiary. I think private insurance policies will be limited to the people who perceive that they have a direct need, which leads to all kinds of adverse selection problems that you would not get under the Rother scheme, which would be universal.

The other point is that if we are going to deal with this as a societal responsibility, we have to look at a system that contemplates participation by the individual, the employer, and society at large in terms of some kind of government effort, both federal and state.

Ms. SCHAEFFER: The point at which coverage really becomes unaffordable does not happen as early as you may think, but it does happen for people 70 years old and beyond.

I find that for people up to age 65, it is quite affordable. You would be surprised at the size of the premium, which I can't quote off the top of my head, but it is affordable.

PART THREE
APPROACHES TO INSURANCE

Part Three examines approaches taken by the private and public sectors to the provision of catastrophic and long-term insurance coverage.

More than half of the U.S. population under 65 had health insurance from an employer-sponsored plan in 1986. Among the nonelderly, the percentage of persons with such coverage was 66 percent. Since the scope of such coverage varies, however, some workers could still face catastrophic out-of-pocket expenses. And despite the extent of employer-provided coverage and the existence of such public programs as Medicare, Medicaid, and the Veterans Administration programs, more than 17 percent of the population reported being without health insurance in 1986.*

In chapter VII, Robert Friedland discusses the different sources of catastrophic health insurance protection and the relative importance of these sources. He then reviews health care expenditures in conjunction with health insurance. Friedland finds that coverage for some types of high-cost health care such as hospital care is relatively common, although hospital care still represents 12.6 percent of total out-of-pocket expenses for the nonelderly. Care provided at hospitals constitutes about 45 percent of personal health care expenditures, Friedland says.

Congress has attempted to assist access to health insurance, through legislation such as the health care continuation provisions of the Consolidated Omnibus Budget Reconciliation Act of 1985 (COBRA). This law requires employers to provide terminated employees and dependents with an opportunity to purchase health insurance from the employers' group plan. Friedland asserts, however, that the law is not likely to fill many of the gaps in coverage, but will increase the cost of providing insurance.

Friedland maintains that attempts to finance catastrophic health care contingencies, including long-term care, through personal savings would be irrational and inefficient, while financing this care through insurance would generally be efficient and within the means

---

*Editor's note: Population includes civilian, nonagricultural workers, nonworkers, and dependents.

of most persons. Access to quality long-term care will become more difficult in the future, Friedland contends, as the number of elderly who need such care increases. Friedland concludes that the public policy debate is likely to focus on how long-term care can be financed through private insurance.

Laurence Lane argues in chapter VIII that the private sector is responding with creative approaches to the demand for long-term care. He divides that response into health-policy oriented and economic-policy oriented approaches.

Under the health policy model, he says, risk factors are tied to specific health status. Financing is through individual or group insurance policies, or long-term disability insurance. Financing and delivery approaches include social health maintenance organizations, life-care communities, and preferred providers.

Under the economic-policy oriented model, Lane says, risk is viewed as a financial condition. One approach is "targeted asset accumulation," which includes efforts to create savings vehicles such as individual medical accounts, to market lump-sum deferred annuities to seniors, or to convert the face value of life insurance products when chronic disability strikes.

Other savings vehicles come under the heading of "untargeted asset accumulation," according to Lane, and include pension and 401(k) asset accumulation, home equity conversion, and life insurance cash values.

The primary vehicle for private financing of long-term care services today, Lane says, is an individual indemnity product. Group insurance coverage for long-term care is a recent development that is gaining momentum. He describes the efforts of several private insurers to market such products.

Lane concludes that considerable progress has been made in recent years to stimulate private market exploration of ways to finance long-term care. More and more insurance companies are weighing the risks of entering the market, he says, although they are proceeding cautiously.

In chapter IX, Janet Myder summarizes the discussion about defining catastrophic health care costs and determining what risks people want to be protected against. Definitions need to consider the out-of-pocket expenditures, individual and family income, and current public or private insurance coverage, she contends.

Myder points out that younger people may also need coverage for long-term care, and older people may incur catastrophic *medical* expenses as well as excessively high long-term care costs. Older people are reasonably well covered for medical expenses, she continues, but not for long-term care costs.

On financing alternatives, Myder asks: "How do we begin or where do we begin?" Judging from poll results, she says, the general public seems to know that we have to spend money, whether public or private, and we must act soon.

In chapter X forum participants discuss the use of Medicaid by the middle class, the willingness of working people to pay for some level of protection, and the role of private insurers and states in providing insurance for long-term care.

VII. Assessing the Need for Catastrophic Health Care Cost Insurance

PAPER BY ROBERT B. FRIEDLAND

Introduction

Health policy discussions in Congress have refocused attention on access to health care, health insurance coverage, and catastrophic health care costs. Given a variety of different circumstances, these issues have taken on new meaning and import. The scope of the debate surrounding these issues has broadened to include low-technology rehabilitation and long-term care assistance in addition to technologically intensive medicine and organ transplants. Furthermore, initiated by health payer "prudent purchasing," profound changes in the financing and delivery of medical care have occurred. These changes have increased the consequences of uncompensated health care for providers and for society and are likely to hinder access to health care for individuals without adequate health insurance.

The health care system now emerging will be severely tested as the number of elderly persons increases (both in absolute and relative terms). Persons age 85 or older will dominate the growth in the U.S. population over the next 25 years as their number more than doubles. In the subsequent 20 years (2010 to 2030) the U.S. population will be dominated by the growth in the relatively young elderly (age 65 to 75). These demographic changes will impact the financing of public health care programs, the demand for health care services, and the cost of these services.[1]

To contain rising health care costs, employers, insurers, and public programs have been encouraged to initiate a variety of changes in plan design, benefits, and reimbursement. These changes in financing have, in turn, elicited complex but pervasive changes in the organization and delivery of health care (Friedland, 1987). As a consequence, having public or private health insurance has become tantamount to having access to health care. Without health insurance, individuals

---

[1]Children born today will be entering the labor force about the time the baby-boom generation is likely to begin retiring. Unless fertility rates change dramatically, the number of persons retiring will be growing faster than the number of new entrants into the labor market.

can face delays in obtaining care and even outright refusal of care. Yet, private or public insurance does not guarantee access to needed health care. Variations in the scope and depth of health insurance coverage may encourage providers to prefer patients with specific types of coverage.

Demographic change and changes in the health care market provide the backdrop from which this paper seeks to assess the relative need for catastrophic and long-term health care coverage for both the elderly and the nonelderly. The paper is divided into three broad sections. The first section discusses the different sources of catastrophic health insurance protection and the relative importance of these sources. Data from the March 1987 Current Population Survey (CPS) are used to examine the extent of health insurance coverage. The second section reviews health care expenditures in conjunction with health insurance. It draws on data from several sources, including the 1980 National Medical Care Utilization and Expenditure Survey (NMCUES), the 1982 Long-Term Care Survey, the 1984 Survey of Income and Program Participation (SIPP), the 1985 National Nursing Home Survey, and the Health Care Financing Administration. The last section draws from the first two sections to assess the need for catastrophic and long-term care insurance. In particular, chronic disability and the ability to pay for uninsured health care are examined using data from SIPP. The last section ends with a brief discussion of recent congressional responses to the issues raised.

Catastrophic Health Care and Health Insurance Coverage

Defining Catastrophic Health Care Expenses—The term "catastrophe" refers to an event or episode that is financially ruinous, suggesting that personal resources are reduced and the individual and his or her family must significantly alter their standard of living. If the goal of public policy is to provide financial protection for families with a member who is in need of medical attention, then catastrophic health care expenditures must be defined in terms of the ability to pay for health care. The ability to pay for needed health care has to do both with the absolute cost of the care and with the patient's financial situation.

Defining catastrophic health care expenditures as out-of-pocket expenditures above some absolute threshold, rather than in terms of ability to pay, changes the relative number and the distribution of persons who would be considered to have had catastrophic expenditures. The size and distribution of the population likely to have catastrophic out-of-pocket expenditures might suggest different public policy options (Wyszewianski, 1986; Berki 1986; Chollet and Betley, 1987). Defining catastrophic health care expenditures in terms of absolute out-of-pocket expenditures would suggest that more than one-third of families with health care expenditures in excess of $2,000 had family incomes in excess of four times the poverty level (table VII.1). If catastrophic expenditures are defined as out-of-pocket health care expenditures in excess of 10 percent of family income (as a measure of ability to pay), only 4.1 percent of families with income four times the poverty level would be considered to have had catastrophic health care expenditures.[2]

Regardless of the definition used, for acute and ambulatory care, persons with "catastrophic" health care expenditures are more likely to be under age 65 (table VII.1). More than 71 percent of all individuals with out-of-pocket expenditures in excess of 10 percent of family income had incomes within 200 percent of poverty—most of these persons (75 percent) were under age 65. Almost 89 percent of all individuals with out-of-pocket expenditures in excess of 10 percent of family income had incomes within 300 percent of poverty in 1980. By comparison, using an absolute dollar threshold, 49 percent of individuals with out-of-pocket expenses in excess of $2,000 had family incomes within 300 percent of poverty.

In addition to changing the distribution of persons with catastrophic expenditures, the particular definition can dramatically alter the number of persons considered to have had catastrophic out-of-pocket expenses for health care. Using $2,000 instead of 10 percent of family income as a definition of the number with catastrophic expenses, raises the number by nearly 11 million. Using 10 percent of family income indicates slightly more elderly (634,875 more) but a lot fewer nonelderly (nearly 12 million fewer) had catastrophic out-of-pocket health care expenditures.

Although three-quarters or more (depending on the definition) of persons with catastrophic out-of-pocket expenditures were under age 65 in 1980, the incidence of catastrophic expenditures is substantially greater among the elderly when ability to pay is used to define catastrophic health care expenditures. Over 15 percent of persons age 65 or older in 1980 had out-of-pocket expenditures for health care in

---

[2]Using out-of-pocket health care expenditures as a percent of income as the measure of ability to pay can be misleading. To assess the family's ability to pay may necessitate evaluating income during and after the episode of care as well as assets and family size.

93

TABLE VII.1
Distribution of Persons with Catastrophic Out-of-Pocket Expenditures under Different Definitions, by Age, 1980[a]

Age	Number of Persons (millions)	Below Poverty[b]	Percentage of Poverty Level 100% to 200%	200% to 300%	300% to 400%	More than 400%	Total
			Out-of-pocket expenditures over $2,000[c]				
Under 65	22.3	6.19%	16.50%	17.95%	15.76%	30.75%	87.16%
Over 65	3.3	0.82	3.38	3.70	2.20	2.75	12.84
Total	25.6	7.01	19.88	21.66	17.96	33.50	100.00
			Out-of-pocket expenditures over 5 percent of family income				
Under 65	27.9	18.54%	25.38%	17.86%	8.00%	6.68%	76.46%
Over 65	8.6	4.83	10.05	5.33	2.09	1.24	23.54
Total	36.5	23.37	35.43	23.20	10.08	7.92	100.00
			Out-of-pocket expenditures over 10 percent of family income				
Under 65	10.9	27.72%	25.61%	11.71%	5.23%	3.19%	73.46%
Over 65	3.9	6.86	11.16	5.47	2.19	0.86	26.54
Total	14.8	34.58	36.77	17.18	7.42	4.05	100.00
			Out-of-pocket expenditures over 20 percent of family income				
Under 65	4.4	43.43%	25.45%	3.76%	1.65%	0.74%	75.04%
Over 65	1.5	10.30	10.91	2.08	1.67	0.00	24.96
Total	5.9	53.74	36.36	5.85	3.32	0.74	100.00

Source: EBRI tabulations of the 1980 National Medical Expenditures Survey.
[a]Excludes institutional nursing home and community-based long-term care.
[b]Poverty income is adjusted for age and family size. For example, in 1980, poverty income for a family of four was $8,414; $4,290 for a nonelderly single individual; and $3,949 for an elderly individual.
[c]The $2,000 dollar threshold is in 1986 dollars. Tabulations are based on the value of this threshold in 1980.

excess of 10 percent of family income; less than 5.4 percent of persons under age 65 were in a similar circumstance. Using $2,000 in annual out-of-pocket expenditures as a threshold of catastrophic health care expenditures, the incidence was 13 percent among the elderly and 11 percent among those under age 65.

Ability to finance necessary health care depends on both how health care is financed and on our ability to pay for care not covered by a health insurance plan. More than 84.4 percent of all persons in the United States have some type of health insurance, but 15.6 percent do not (table VII.2). For the 37.4 million people without health insurance, ability to pay determines the amount of health care that is catastrophic. For the 201.4 million persons with health insurance, the breath and depth of their insurance coverage generally reduces the financial aftermath of health care; ability to pay becomes secondary. The wider the scope of services covered and the deeper the coverage, the less likely any particular covered service will be financially devastating.

Catastrophic Coverage Provided by Employer Plans—Employer-provided health plans are the primary source of health insurance coverage in the United States, providing more than half (58 percent in 1986) of the U.S. population with health insurance (table VII.2) Sixty-six percent of the nonelderly have employer-provided insurance.[3]

Among families with at least one worker, 80 percent have employer-provided health insurance and if the largest earner in the family was not unemployed during the year, the proportion increases to 85 percent.

The scope of coverage provided by employer-provided health insurance varies; participants, however, might still face catastrophic out-of-pocket expenditures. Sources of out-of-pocket costs for employer-plan participants include uncovered services, copayments, deductibles, and all health care expenses beyond plan maximums. Virtually no one has coverage for long-term care. Although 33 percent of health plan participants in medium and large establishments have coverage for extended care, this is usually for recuperative care in a skilled nursing home or hospice care—not long-term care for a chronic disability. All participants in employer-provided health plans in medium and large establishments have coverage for hospital care, intensive care, outpatient care and diagnostic X-ray and laboratory

---

[3]Unless otherwise noted, all 1986 health insurance coverage figures are from EBRI tabulations of the March 1987 Current Population Survey, U.S. Department of Commerce, Bureau of the Census.

TABLE VII.2
Health Insurance Coverage of the Entire U.S.
Population by Source of Coverage, 1986

	Number (thousands)	Percentage
Total	238,789	100.0%
Employer provided	138,510	58.0
Medicare	25,141	10.5
Medicaid	16,124	6.8
CHAMPUS	8,610	3.6
Medicare and Medicaid	3,379	1.4
Medicare and CHAMPUS	1,105	0.5
Medicaid and CHAMPUS	228	0.1
Other private and public	8,335	3.5
No coverage	37,357	15.6

Source: EBRI tabulations of the March 1987 Current Population Survey, U.S. Bureau of the Census.

Note: May not add to total because of rounding.

services. Some participants have no coverage for physician office visits (4 percent) or prescription drugs (2 percent), but some had these services covered in full (U.S. Department of Labor, 1987).

Copayments and deductibles can, depending on the extent of health care use and family income, become financially burdensome. Most plan participants, however, are in plans that limit out-of-pocket payments for the copayments and deductibles of covered services in any particular year (table VII.3). More than half of the participants were in plans with copayments limited to $1,200 or less and three-quarters participated in plans that limited the out-of-pocket expense for covered services to $2,000 or less.

Generally, plans covering smaller firms included higher out-of-pocket limits than larger firms. Of firms with more than 500 employees, 88 percent limited liabilities to less than $2,000, while 68 percent of firms with fewer than 25 employees limited liabilities to under $2,000 (Employee Benefit Research Institute, 1987). Over half (63 percent) of the workers in medium and large establishments participating in a health plan had a deductible for covered services that was less than $100 in 1987, 31 percent had a deductible of between $100 and $200, and 6 percent had a deductible of more than $200.

While most employer-sponsored health insurance plans limit an employee's out-of-pocket expenses for covered services in any given year, there may be limits on the amount covered over the life of the

TABLE VII.3
Percentage of Full-Time Workers in Medium and Large Firms in Employer-Sponsored Major Medical Plans, with Various Plan Provisions Relating to Participant Cost, 1986

Plan Provision		Percentage of Participants
Plan deductible		
$50 or less		11%
$51 to $100		47
$101 to $150		16
$151 to $200		15
More than $200		6
No deductible		1
Based on earnings		4
Summary: less than $200		94
Plan coinsurance		
Health plan pays all expenses when covered expenses reach	Maximum participant coinsurance[a]	
$2,000	$400	10%
$4,000	$800	22
$6,000	$1,200	30
$8,000	$1,600	6
$10,000	$2,000	9
more than $10,000	greater than $2,000	4
coinsurance reduced or unchanged	unlimited	19
Plan maximum		
Lifetime maximum		
$50,000 or less		4%
$50,001 to $100,000		2
$100,001 to $250,000		19
$250,001 to $500,000		18
Greater than $500,000		25
Lifetime and annual or disability maximum		5
Annual or disability maximum only		7
No maximum		20
Summary		

(continued)

TABLE VII.3 (continued)

Plan Provision	Percentage of Participants
maximum greater than $100,000	82
maximum greater than $250,000	63

Source: U.S. Department of Labor, Bureau of Labor Statistics, *Employee Benefits in Medium and Large Firms, 1986* (Washington DC: U.S. Government Printing Office, 1987) tables 34–36.
[a]Assumes 80 percent copayment. In 1986, 86 percent of employees in medium-size and large establishments who participated in employer-sponsored major medical coverage had plans that paid 80 percent of the cost of covered services after the deductible.

plan. The lifetime maximum benefit varies from $50,000 or less to no such provision for a lifetime maximum. For participants in health insurance plans in medium and large establishments in 1986, 20 percent had no lifetime maximum, 6 percent had lifetime maximums of less than $100,000, and 37 percent had limits of between $100,000 and $500,000.

Catastrophic Coverage Provided by Public Insurance Programs—Three public programs—Medicare, Medicaid, and the Veterans Administration (VA)—finance most health care services. (Beginning in 1989, the scope of coverage and the financing of many Medicare services will change. See Appendix C for a description of these changes.) Eligibility for these programs and the scope and depth of coverage vary. Veterans with service-related disabilities are entitled to care in the VA system (which includes hospitals, nursing homes, and outpatient clinics). Veterans in need of medical assistance who were not disabled in service but who have limited financial means can also obtain access to this system.

In general, Medicare eligibility is conferred on persons age 65 or older who are eligible to receive Social Security benefits; on persons, regardless of age, who have been receiving Social Security disability payments for 24 months; or on persons who have end-stage renal disease. Almost 31 million persons, or nearly 13 percent of the U.S. population, were Medicare beneficiaries and total expenditures were $74.1 billion in 1986 (U.S. Department of Health and Human Services, 1987). Medicare coverage among the noninstitutionalized elderly is over 96 percent and is about 1 percent among the nonelderly.

Sources of out-of-pocket expenditures for Medicare enrollees include services that are not covered, deductibles, copayments, physician charges above what Medicare determines as reasonable, and Part B premiums. There is no premium charged for Part A benefits, but there are deductibles and copayments. In 1988, the hospital deductible (per episode of care) is $540 and the copayment is $135 per day for the 61st through 90th day in the hospital associated with a particular spell of illness. If the stay goes beyond 90 days, the daily copayment is $270. Medicare covered care in a skilled nursing home imposes no deductible, but requires a copayment of $65 a day for days 21 through 100. For Part B coverage there is a monthly premium, annual deductible, and a 20 percent copayment for covered services. The monthly premium for Part B coverage is $24.80 in 1988 and the annual deductible is $75. If the physician does not accept Medicare assignment, charges above the Medicare-determined charge, in addition to the 20 percent copayment, are the patient's responsibility.

Medicaid provides health care for very low-income persons in specific categories. Eligibility requirements are established by each state within broad federal guidelines and are not uniform across states. In 1986, 8.3 percent of the U.S. population had been covered at some time during the year by Medicaid. Although most Medicaid recipients are under age 65, Medicaid is an important source of insurance for the elderly. About 10 percent of the elderly and 3.5 percent of the nonelderly were covered in 1986. Medicaid covered about 40 percent of the poor (or 13.8 million persons) and over 14 percent of the near-poor[4] (1.6 million persons).

In general, low-income families qualify for Medicaid either as "categorically needy" or "medically needy." States must cover those who are categorically needy—people who qualify for cash assistance under the Aid to Families with Dependent Children (AFDC) program or the Supplemental Security Income (SSI) program for the aged, blind, and disabled.[5] At their option, states may also cover the medically needy: people who would qualify for either AFDC or the SSI program except that (1) their income levels are slightly above the categorically needy program standard but below the medically needy standard[6] or (2) their income is higher than the medically needy standard but falls below it after subtracting medical expenses (over a specific pe-

---

[4]Near poor is defined as those with family income between the federal poverty income standard and 125 percent of that standard.
[5]Technically, receipt of SSI payments is a necessary requirement but not a sufficient criterion for Medicaid eligibility. Fourteen states [the 209(b) states] use more restrictive rules than the federal SSI standard. In 1986, the federal SSI income standard was $336 a month for a single individuals and $504 for a couple; countable assets could not exceed $1,700 for individuals and $2,550 for couples.
[6]A monthly income amount between the AFDC standard and 133⅓ percent of this standard. The actual standard across states varies from $108 to $475 a month for single persons (Tilly and Bruner, 1987, table 4).

riod of time.)[7] Thirty-eight states cover the medically needy. In addition, states have the option of including specific "state-only" eligibility groups of low-income persons who receive cash assistance from the state but are not categorically eligible for AFDC or SSI.

By federal law, Medicaid must provide hospital care, physician services, and skilled nursing care; but states may also include coverage for drugs, intermediate nursing home care, and dental services. States can impose a nominal copayment for the optional benefits, but most do not and of those that do (22 in 1984) in no case was it more than $3.00 per service (Howell et al., 1985). In 1985, there were 21.8 million recipients of Medicaid and total state and federal expenditures for services totaled $39 billion. Hospital and nursing home care are the two largest sources of Medicaid expenditures; together they account for three-quarters of program costs. More than 37 percent of expenditures were for hospital care and 37 percent was for nursing home care.

Persons without Health Insurance—In 1986, more than 15 percent of the U.S. population reported that they were without health insurance. Although some of these 37.4 million people without insurance are uninsured only part of the time, some 20 to 25 million individuals seem to be permanently without coverage (Reinhardt, 1987). Previous work, concentrating on the nonelderly population, has demonstrated three salient facts about the uninsured.[8] First, more than three-quarters (77.5 percent) of the uninsured in 1986 were employed or the dependents of workers. About one-half of the uninsured were in families headed by someone who worked full-time all year. Second, most of the uninsured workers have relatively low earnings. In 1985, more than 69 percent of uninsured workers earned less than $10,000 and nearly 92 percent earned less than $20,000 (EBRI, 1987). Finally, uninsured workers tend to be located in smaller firms primarily in the service sectors. In 1983, 38.2 percent of uninsured workers were in firms of less than 25 employees, and 27.3 percent were self-em-

---

[7]This is the spend-down test. To become eligible, an individual's income, medical expenses, and assets are examined over a period of time that varies by state from one to six months. If during that time the individual qualifies, then the person is determined eligible for Medicaid (until the test is repeated). After becoming eligible, a separate calculation is done to determine how much the individual will have to contribute toward his or her care.

[8]Most of EBRI's work on the nonelderly population excludes those in the military or in agricultural work. For more information on this issue, see Employee Benefit Research Institute, *EBRI Issue Brief* 58 (September 1986); *EBRI Issue Brief* 62 (January 1987); and *EBRI Issue Brief* 66 (May 1987).

ployed. More than 50 percent of the uninsured workers were in retail trade or other services (EBRI, 1987).

More than one-half of the uninsured (61 percent) were in families with family income that was less than twice the federal poverty income level (table VII.4). About one-third of the uninsured were in families with incomes that were below poverty. Nearly 35 percent of all persons with family incomes below poverty (14.4 percent of the population), were without health insurance in 1986; 65.3 percent, however, had either public or private health insurance (table VII.4). The single largest source, Medicaid, covered 40 percent of the very poor; while employers covered 11 percent and Medicare covered less than 8 percent. Persons with family income between the poverty standard and twice the poverty standard (19 percent of the population) were more likely to have private insurance coverage and less likely to have public health insurance coverage. Medicaid accounted for about 30 percent, Medicare accounted for 10 percent and employers accounted for nearly 41 percent of the health insurance coverage in this group. By comparison, among the one-third of the U.S. population with family incomes four times the poverty standard or greater, health insurance coverage is 93 percent, 80 percent of which is from private insurance.

Health Care Utilization and Expenditures

In general, we tend to incur more medical expenses as we grow older. Old age brings with it a greater propensity for aches, pains, and illnesses that encourage physician visits, hospitalizations, diagnostic testing, and other procedures. Medications are increasingly needed as are medical devices such as hearing aids, eye-glasses, canes, walkers, and wheel-chairs. But these expenses are relatively small compared to the expense of a hospital stay that may require intensive use of life-sustaining technology.

Proximity to death is a major cause of high expenditures. Heroic efforts to thwart respiratory or heart failure, for example, are very expensive. Fuchs has estimated that more than 1 percent of GNP is consumed on health expenditures by persons in their last year of life (Fuchs, 1984). Consequently, the elderly use a disproportionate share of health services. In 1984, the elderly represented 12 percent of the population but consumed more than 35 percent of all health care expenditures (table VII.5). On a per capita basis, health expenditures

TABLE VII.4
Health Insurance Coverage by Source and Distribution, by Family Income as a Percentage of Poverty Level, 1986

	Percentage of Poverty Level							
	Less than 100%		100%–199%		200%–399%		Greater than 400%	
	Number (thousands)	Percentage	Number (thousands)	Percentage	Number (thousands)	Percentage	Number (thousands)	Percentage
Private only	5,439	15.8%	20,863	46.3%	59,162	71.5%	61,343	80.2%
Public only	15,008	43.5	7,754	17.2	5,603	6.8	2,630	3.4
Public and private	2,046	5.9	5,605	12.4	8,777	10.6	7,202	9.4
Total with coverage	22,492	65.3	34,221	75.0	73,542	88.8	71,175	93.1
Total without coverage	11,974	34.7	10,832	24.0	9,254	11.2	5,297	6.9

Source EBRI tabulations of the March 1987 Current Population Survey, U.S. Department of Commerce, Bureau of the Census.
Note: Poverty income is adjusted for family size and age. For example, poverty income for a family of four in 1986 was $11,203; $5,701 for a single nonelderly person; and $5,225 for a single elderly person.

TABLE VII.5

Health Care Expenditures by Source and as a Percentage of Total Health Care Expenditures among the Elderly and Nonelderly, 1984

	Under Age 65		Age 65 and Older	
Source of Care	Spending (billions)	Percentage of total spending	Spending (billions)	Percentage of total spending
Hospital	$103.7	30.3%	$ 54.2	15.9%
Nursing homes	6.9	2.0	25.1	7.3
Physicians	50.6	14.8	24.8	7.2
Other	60.7	17.8	15.8	4.6
Total	221.9	64.9	119.9	35.1

Source: EBRI tabulations from Levit, Katherine R., Helen Lazenby, Daniel R. Waldo, and Lawrence M. Davidoff, "National Health Expenditures, 1984," *Health Care Financing Review* 1 (Fall 1985), table 2; and Waldo, Daniel, and Helen Lazenby, "Demographic Characteristics and Health Care Use and Expenditures by the Aged in the United States: 1977–1984," *Health Care Financing Review* 1 (Fall 1984), table 11.

in 1984 were nearly four times greater for persons over age 65 ($4,202 per person) than for persons under age 65 ($1,211 per person).[9]

In terms of expenditures, hospitals serve as the largest single source of health care received by both the elderly and the nonelderly. Care provided at hospitals constitutes about 45 percent of personal health care expenditures; in 1984, the elderly consumed nearly 16 percent and the nonelderly consumed 30 percent of total personal health care expenditures on hospital care. For the elderly, the second largest provider of health care is nursing homes, while for the nonelderly it is from dental care, drugs, medical sundries, appliances, and other professional and personal health care services combined.

Sources of Catastrophic Expenditures—Out-of-pocket expenditures reflect services that are less likely to be covered by insurance. Most of the elderly (98 percent) have Medicare and most Medicare beneficiaries (72 percent) have supplemental Medigap coverage. Consequently, out-of-pocket expenditures for acute care and ambulatory care in the aggregate are relatively small for the elderly. Hospital care for the elderly represented 1.8 percent of total out-of-pocket spending, and physician care represented less than 7 percent (table VII.6). For the nonelderly, hospital care represented 12.6 percent of

---

[9]Author's calculation of National Health Expenditure data published in Levit, et al., 1985, table 2, and Waldo and Lazenby, 1984, table 11.

TABLE VII.6
Distribution of Out-of-Pocket Expenditures for Health Care by Age, 1984

| | Under Age 65 | | Age 65 and Older | |
Source of Care	Spending (billions)	Percentage of total spending	Spending (billions)	Percentage of total out-of-pocket spending
Hospital	$12.0	12.6%	$ 1.7	1.8%
Nursing homes	3.2	3.4	12.6	13.2
Physicians	14.5	15.2	6.5	6.8
Other	35.5	37.2	9.5	9.9
Total	65.3	68.3	30.2	31.6

Source: EBRI tabulations from Levit, Katherine R., Helen Lazenby, Daniel R. Waldo, and Lawrence M. Davidoff, "National Health Expenditures, 1984," *Health Care Financing Review* 1 (Fall 1985), table 2; and Waldo, Daniel, and Helen Lazenby, "Demographic Characteristics and Health Care Use and Expenditures by the Aged in the United States: 1977–1984," *Health Care Financing Review* 1 (Fall 1984), table 11.

total out-of-pocket expenditures and physician care represented over 15 percent. These differences between the elderly and the nonelderly reflect, in part, the near universal health insurance coverage through Medicare and Medigap policies among the elderly and the greater likelihood that this coverage is more comprehensive for acute and ambulatory care.

The distribution of out-of-pocket expenses can differ significantly by source of insurance coverage (table VII.7). These differences, however, reflect both the health status of the insured and the scope of coverage. Overall, the average total charge per capita was $730, of which 27 percent was paid out-of-pocket. The elderly had total mean per capita charges nearly three times that of the nonelderly, but out-of-pocket expenditures as a percentage of total charges were less (19 percent as opposed to 30 percent). Although the elderly had a relatively smaller exposure to total charges, the average per capita out-of-pocket expense was greater owing to the greater charges. On average, the per capita out-of-pocket expenses of the elderly were almost twice that of the nonelderly ($327 versus $179).

Medicare coverage, if not supplemented with additional coverage, however, leaves both the elderly and the nonelderly at greatest risk for catastrophic health care expenditures. Among the nonelderly, mean per capita out-of-pocket expenses were the least for those with Medicaid and the most for those with Medicare (without Medicaid). This

Mean Per Capita Charges and Out-of-Pocket Expense, Percentage of Total Charges Paid Out-of-Pocket, and Coverage for Noninstitutionalized Persons, by Age and Type of Health Insurance Coverage: United States, 1980

Age and Type of Coverage	Mean per Capita Total Charge	Mean per Capita Out-of-Pocket Expense	Percentage of Total Charges Paid Out-of-Pocket	Persons Covered Number in millions	Persons Covered Percent
All persons	$730	$195	27	217.9	—
Under 65 years of age					
Total	604	179	30	194.0	100.0
Medicaid	766	72	9	18.1	9.3
Medicare, no Medicaid	2,542	441	17	2.2	1.2
Private, no Medicaid or Medicare	615	192	31	141.8	73.1
Other coverage	695	107	15	5.9	3.0
No coverage	218	179	82	25.8	13.3
65 years of age or over					
Total	1,760	327	19	23.8	100.0
Medicare only	1,104	319	29	4.9	20.5
Medicare and Medicaid	3,106	233	7	2.9	12.2
Medicare and other coverage	1,767	352	20	15.1	63.5
Other coverage	903	195	22	0.6	2.7
No coverage	a	a	67	a	a

Source: Howell, Embry, Larry Corder, and Allen Dobson, "Out-of-Pocket Health Expenses for Medicaid Recipients and Low-Income Persons, 1980," in National Medical Care Utilization and Expenditures Survey, U.S. Department of Health and Human Services, Office of Research and Demonstrations, Series B, Descriptive Report no. 4 (Washington, D.C.: U.S. Government Printing Office, 1985).

[a]Sample too small for accurate estimate.

reflects the fact that the nonelderly with Medicare are likely, by virtue of their disabilities, to be heavy users of health care and because Medicaid provides relatively broad and deep coverage. Average per person out-of-pocket expenses among those with private insurance only were less than one-half that of those with Medicare—but as a percentage of total charges were much greater. This difference may reflect the relatively healthy nature of the privately insured population and greater cost-sharing or relatively less coverage for routine ambulatory health care among the privately insured population.

Among the elderly, average out-of-pocket expenditures per person were about the same, regardless of the source of coverage. However, those with Medicare and Medicaid (the "dually eligible") paid the smallest percent of out-of-pocket and those with Medicare alone paid the largest. The dually eligible are, in general, in very ill health (McMillan et al., 1983; McMillan and Gornick, 1984); but their Medicaid and Medicare coverage provides broad and deep insurance protection. Those with Medicare alone face cost sharing often paid by Medigap policies or employer-provided retiree health benefits.

Relatively few persons are intensive users of health care. Differences among individuals therefore are not appropriately captured in per capita averages. In 1984, only 15 percent of the population age 45 or older had had a hospitalization.[10] In 1980, about 5 percent of all persons had no out-of-pocket health expenditures for health care. Nearly 83 percent of all persons had out-of-pocket health expenditures of 5 percent or less of family income; 4.2 percent had 15 percent or more and 7.2 percent had 11 percent or more. Nearly 85 percent of the nonelderly spent 5 percent of their family income or less on health care, and less than 4 percent spent more than 15 percent of their income. More than one-third of the elderly spent 6 percent or more of their family income on health care, and 10 percent spent more than 15 percent.

The mean per capita out-of-pocket health care expenses (except nursing home costs) for all noninstitutionalized persons with health care expenditures was $246 in 1980. Among persons under age 65 the average was $229 and for persons over age 65 it was $370 (tables VII.8 and VII.9). The largest source of out-of-pocket expenses for both the elderly and the nonelderly was for hospital care. Mean per capita expenses for this care were relatively similar: $669 for the nonelderly and $710 for the elderly. For the nonelderly without health insurance,

---

[10] Preliminary EBRI tabulations of Survey of Income and Program Participation (SIPP), U.S. Department of Commerce, Bureau of the Census.

TABLE VII.8

Mean Per Capita Out-of-Pocket Expenses for Persons under 65 Years of Age with Expense, by Health Insurance Coverage and Type of Service: United States, 1980

Type of Service	All Persons	Total	Private, No Medicare, No Medicaid	Medicaid	Medicare, No Medicaid	Other Coverage	No Coverage
Total	$245.82	$228.66	$225.32	$ 169.17	$482.15	$168.21	$ 255.31
Dental visit	111.25	107.54	103.05	92.87	87.22	119.28	106.49
Orthodontia visit	462.81	465.22	463.55	a	a	a	a
Doctor's office visit	76.02	72.76	72.31	64.21	99.24	65.19	75.62
Emergency room visit	58.03	59.51	50.76	63.75	a	49.92	89.76
Out-patient visit	69.04	67.59	62.05	98.58	74.86	57.04	91.98
Other medical provider visit	79.05	80.13	81.66	71.64	63.55	66.37	74.66
Hospital stay	678.29	669.38	560.47	1,059.69	987.57	229.71	1,380.13
Prescribed medicine	42.24	34.03	32.51	27.66	124.88	32.02	33.39
Other medical expense	76.06	72.51	71.72	66.86	78.77	80.75	81.76

Note: [a] Sample too small for accurate estimate.

Source: Howell, Embry, Larry Corder, and Allen Dobson, "Out-of-Pocket Health Expenses for Medicaid Recipients and Low-Income Persons, 1980," in *National Medical Care Utilization and Expenditures Survey*, U.S. Department of Health and Human Services, Office of Research and Demonstrations, Series B, Descriptive Report no. 4 (Washington, D.C.: U.S. Government Printing Office, 1985).

TABLE VII.9
Mean Per Capita Out-of-Pocket Expenses for Persons 65 Years of Age or Over with Expense, by Health Insurance Coverage and Type of Service: United States, 1980.

Type of Service	All Persons	Total	Total Medicare	Medicare Only	Medicare and Medicaid	Medicare and Other Coverage	Private and Other Insurance
Total	$245.82	$369.47	$370.23	$380.13	$301.21	$378.47	$256.63
Dental visit	111.25	147.51	148.22	153.39	153.41	149.08	114.8
Orthodontia visit	462.81	a	a	a	a	a	a
Doctor's office visit	76.02	97.22	97.57	97.56	86.95	98.63	96.29
Emergency room visit	58.03	43.84	44.21	57.90	a	41.44	a
Out-patient visit	69.04	77.13	76.57	53.61	a	85.89	a
Other medical provider visit	79.05	72.28	73.19	96.21	54.10	69.51	a
Hospital stay	678.29	710.04	708.94	769.99	1,204.04	599.64	a
Prescribed medicine	42.24	89.31	89.75	98.17	43.22	94.91	74.18
Other medical expense	76.06	90.43	89.85	78.94	68.00	93.08	a

Source: Howell, Embry, Larry Corder, and Allen Dobson, "Out-of-Pocket Health Expenses for Medicaid Recipients and Low-Income Persons, 1980," in *National Medical Care Utilization and Expenditures Survey*, U.S. Department of Health and Human Services, Office of Research and Demonstrations, Series B, Descriptive Report No. 4 (Washington, D.C.: U.S. Government Printing Office, 1985).

aSample too small for accurate estimate.

the mean per capita out-of-pocket hospital costs ($1,380) were more than twice the average (Table VII.8). For persons with Medicaid, out-of-pocket costs for hospital care were more than one and a half times the average ($1,059). Among the elderly with a hospital visit, mean per capita out-of-pocket expenditures for the dually eligible (Medicare and Medicaid) were also more than one and a half times the average ($1,204; table VII.9) For the nonelderly, the second largest source of out-of-pocket expenditures was for orthodontia care; while for the elderly it was dental care.

Medicare, however, does not cover long-term nursing home care. Consequently, nursing homes represent the elderly's single largest source of out-of-pocket expenses. In 1984, nursing home expenditures on behalf of the elderly were $32 billion—Medicare paid $0.6 billion and private insurance paid $0.3 billion. Most of the remainder was shared directly from out-of-pocket expenditures ($15.8 billion) and Medicaid ($13.9 billion). Care in a skilled nursing home ranges from $58 to $80 a day, and care in a intermediate care facility ranges from $44 to $63 a day (Strahan, 1987). This places the cost of nursing home care at around $1,800 a month. Although many persons enter nursing homes for a relatively short period of time, among long-time residents, the duration can be many years. Overall, the median length of stay among residents in 1985 was over 20 months (Hing, 1987).

By including nursing home costs, the relative importance of hospital care as a major source of out-of-pocket expenditures is reduced. In the aggregate, nursing home expenditures are the elderly's largest source of out-of-pocket expenses. Of total out-of-pocket expenditures among the elderly, nearly 13 percent was spent for nursing home care in 1984, while less than 2 percent was spent out-of-pocket for hospital care (table VII.6). Among all elderly with health care expenditures of $2,000 or more, over 81 percent of the out-of-pocket expenses were estimated to be for nursing home care, while 10 percent were for hospital care (Rice and Gabel, 1986).

Assessing the Need for Catastrophic and Long-Term Care Insurance

Coverage for some types of high cost health care (in particular hospital care) is relatively common. Nearly all persons, however, are without insurance that covers care in a nursing home or the assistance of an aide, nurse, or therapist (physical, speech, occupational) who provides care in one's home.[11] Although certain high cost acute care procedures may be financially catastrophic, among the nonelderly insured population the uncovered areas of care are the most expensive (orthodontia, dental care, and long-term care). For the elderly, long-term care is clearly the greatest financial concern. At any point in time, 5 percent of the elderly are in nursing homes and another 16 percent need some level of assistance to remain in the community. Average out-of-pocket expenditures among the disabled elderly in the community for long-term care were $164 per month in 1982, but for the most severely limited the average was $439 (Lui, et al., 1986). For victims of Alzheimer's disease, the monthly cost of care at home can exceed $1,200 (Lien-Fu Huang, et al., 1985). Care in a nursing home is only a portion of what is generally referred to as long-term care. Long-term care is an array of health care, personal care, and social services delivered over a sustained (but not necessarily continuous) period to persons who have lost or never acquired some degree of functional capacity. In 1986, national expenditures on nursing homes exceeded $38 billion. More than 50 percent or $19.4 billion was paid directly out-of-pocket. Estimates for 1985 suggest that nursing home care represents about 72 percent of all formal long-term care (Chollet and Friedland, forthcoming).

Not everyone will need long-term care. In 1984, 16 percent of the noninstitutionalized population reported some level of disability and about 7.5 percent of the noninstitutionalized population age 15 or older reported needing the assistance of another person (table VII.10). Most of the population with relatively servere disabilities, however, were age 45 or older. Nearly 2 million children under age 15 and over 2 million young adults (less than age 25) report functional limitations (U.S. Department of Commerce, 1986). However, more than one-half the persons age 15 or older reporting relatively severe limitations were age 70 or older and over 86 percent were age 55 or older. Among individuals age 75 or older, 41 percent were severely limited.

Presumably, nursing home residents would also be considered severely limited. In 1985, there were nearly 1.5 million nursing home residents (Strahan, 1987). Most residents were elderly, but 2.5 percent

---

[11]The market for private long-term care insurance is growing, however. The U.S. Department of Health and Human Services Task Force on Long-Term Health Care Policies estimates that as of May 1987 there were 73 companies selling policies and that 422,691 policies had been sold. In addition, the State of Alaska now offers access to a long-term care policy for retirees and their dependents. Between March and October 1987, one-third of the state of Alaska retirees and their spouses had enrolled (2,276 retirees and 973 spouses).

TABLE VII.10
Prevalence of Relatively Severe Disability among the Noninstitutionalized Population Age 15 and Older, 1984 (thousands)

Age Group	Total Population	Severe Limitations[a]	Percent among the Disabled	Percent within Each Age Group
Total	180,987	13,536	100.0%	7.48%
15-24	39,297	346	2.6	0.88
25-34	40,464	596	4.4	1.47
35-44	30,480	890	6.6	2.92
45-54	22,264	1,431	10.6	6.43
55-64	22,060	2,734	20.2	12.39
65-69	8,928	1,682	12.4	18.84
70-74	7,378	1,691	12.5	22.92
75+	10,116	4,166	41.2	41.18

Source: EBRI tabulations of Survey of Income and Program Participation (SIPP) data, U.S. Department of Commerce, Bureau of the Census, 1986.

[a]Severe limitation is based on the need for assistance from another person in doing either light housework, preparing meals, dressing, eating, personal hygiene, or getting around.

were under 45 years of age and 11 percent were age 45 to 64. More than one-half (54.8 percent) of all nursing home residents, however, were age 80 or older, and 80 percent were age 70 or older (U.S. Department of Health and Human Services, 1987).

Estimates of the lifetime risk of entering a nursing home vary, but one recent study estimates that the lifetime risk at age 65 is 30 percent for men and 52 percent for women (Cohen et al., 1986). In their study, the risk for women is estimated to peak at 57 percent at age 79, while for men the risk peaks at 31 percent at age 74.

The ability of a person with a debilitating condition to stay in the community is in large part dependent on informal care from family (and friends) and the availability of certain community-based social services, but it is also based on the ability to liquidate assets to pay for care. Those with the most severe chronic limitations are, in general, the least likely to have the ability to pay for health care. The findings in table VII.11 suggest that persons who are most severely limited still living in the community might have ample income, but have virtually no assets. Median net wealth and income among the population (age 45 or older) free from chronic disabilities was twice that of persons reporting a relatively mild limitation in 1984 (table VII.11). Persons with at least one very serious limitation in activities

111

TABLE VII.11
Average Age, Income, and Wealth of the U.S. Population Age 45 and Older by Levels of Disability

Level of Assistance	Average Age	Median Net Wealth	Median Income	Percent of Persons
None	61	$13,250	$8,810	81.3%
Limited[a]	68	6,250	5,890	15.4
Some[b]	70	634	5,207	2.0
More[c]	82	13	4,656	0.5
Most[d]	73	0	5,864	0.9

Source: Preliminary EBRI tabulations of the Survey of Income and Program Participation (SIPP) data, U.S. Department of Commerce, 1984.

[a] Difficulty getting around outside the house without assistance, help needed to do light housework, prepare meals, and lift more than 10 pounds.
[b] Either needs assistance from someone to get around inside the house, transfer into or out of bed, or needs help with personal needs (dressing, undressing, eating, or personal hygiene).
[c] Assistance is needed for personal needs and assistance either with transferring or moving about.
[d] Assistance is needed with personal needs, transferring, and mobility.

necessary to live from day to day (over 1.4 million people) had one-tenth of the net wealth of the mildly limited group and were, on average, only slightly older. Among the nearly one million people with two or three serious limitations in activities necessary for daily living, median wealth was negligible but median family income was $5,585.

Congressional Response—Congress has responded to some of the issues related to the uninsured, and some of the catastrophic health care expenses faced by the elderly. In the Consolidated Omnibus Budget Reconciliation Act of 1985 (COBRA, P.L. 99-272), workers and their dependents who might lose health insurance coverage from a either a change in employment or marital status were provided the opportunity to purchase health insurance from the employer's group plan for 18 to 36 months (depending on the circumstance).

Although a deliberate attempt to assist access to health insurance, the health care continuation provisions in COBRA are not likely to fill many of the gaps in coverage. Most of the uninsured are either employees or dependents of workers who work in firms that do not offer health insurance. Secondly, although employer-group health insurance plans tend to be more comprehensive than individually purchased policies, they are also likely to be more expensive, making it difficult for many eligible workers to afford coverage.

On the face of it, there is at least one recent change in the 1986 tax reform bill (P.L. 99-514) that could interpret congressional intentions quite differently from those in COBRA continuation provisions. Prior to tax reform, individual health care expenses above 5 percent of adjusted gross income could be deducted from taxable income. Now, health care expenses are not deductible until they exceed 7.5 percent of adjusted gross income. Given the change in marginal tax rates, individuals with high out-of-pocket expenses might not be any worse off (in terms of tax liability) after tax reform. However, this assumes that individual tax liabilities after tax reform are lower and that marginal tax rates are not increased in the future.

The COBRA's continuation provisions, in conjunction with the new nondiscrimination rules on employer-provided health insurance plans imposed by tax reform, tend to increase the cost of providing health insurance. Raising the cost of health insurance might inhibit new firms from offering health insurance, especially in sectors where the likelihood of receiving health insurance coverage is already low and the ability to attract workers may not depend on providing health benefits. As the cost of providing health insurance increases, the threshold at which new firms would find it financially advantageous (or even feasible) to provide health insurance benefits is raised. For firms already providing health insurance, if benefits become too expensive, the use of part-time or contractual workers could become an increasingly attractive alternative.

Finally, Congress is considering recommendations from the HHS Task Force on Long Term Health Care Policies to facilitate the private market for long-term care insurance.* In particular, the task force has recommended favorable clarification in the tax code for insurance reserves, premiums, and benefits, and has also proposed that individuals be allowed to draw on pension funds to finance long-term care premiums.

Concluding Comments

Poor health, diseases, accidents, and disabilities are not confined to specific groups of individuals. By and large, these events are distributed unevenly across the population and, for any individual, unevenly over his or her lifetime.[12] Without health insurance, all but a

---

*Editor's note: see Appendix B.

[12] In all likelihood there is a positive correlation between poor health and income, since persons with low income (and no health insurance) avoid preventive health care, and many persons with poor health are unable to work.

very few persons might find most ambulatory, acute, or long-term care costs associated with serious illness or injury financially catastrophic. Saving for these contingencies is both irrational and inefficient. Financing this care through insurance, on the other hand, is generally efficient and within the means of most persons (Chollet and Friedland, 1988).

The risk of needing assistance in activities necessary for daily living increases with age. Consequently, increases in the number of elderly (in particular the number age 85 or older) virtually ensures that without significant reductions in the prevalence of debilitating conditions, the number of elderly who will need assistance will increase. Manton and Liu (1984) estimate that the number of elderly with limitations in activities of daily living (including eating, dressing, moving to or from a bed to a chair, using the toilet, for example) or instrumental activities of daily living (including preparing meals, shopping, managing money, light housekeeping, moving about outside) will nearly triple in 60 years, reaching 18.8 million in 2040, if the prevalence of chronic conditions among the elderly remains the same.

These projections suggest that over the next 25 years the demand for institutional long-term care services could increase 73 percent, and the demand for noninstitutional care will increase 66 percent. Increases in demand of this magnitude could put substantial upward pressure on prices for institutional and noninstitutional chronic care services that are now in short supply. As the price increases, access to quality long-term care becomes more difficult.

The public policy debate over the next few years is likely to focus on facilitating the private financing of long-term care. In their search for containing health care costs, employers may want to consider this opportunity to incorporate long-term care into the continuum of health care already covered.[13] Congress may be more inclined, given the size of the federal deficit, to find mechanisms that will encourage the private market. Failure of the private market to develop broad-based protection, however, could lead to a larger public-sector role in the financing of long-term and other catastrophic health care costs.

Everyone is at risk in terms of needing catastrophic and long-term health care. We all must rely on the same health care delivery system. The availability of necessary services now, as well as in the future, is directly related to how we finance our health care.

---

[13]There may be efficiencies in effectively managing both acute and long-term care.

114

References

Berki, S.E. "A Look at Catastrophic Medical Expenses and the Poor." *Health Affairs* 4 (Winter 1986): 138–145.

Chollet, Deborah J., and Charles Betley. "Financing Catastrophic Health Care Among the Nonelderly Population." *Business and Health* 11 (September, 1987).

————, and Robert B. Friedland. "Employer Financing of Long-Term Care." In R. Scheffler and L. Rossiter (eds) *Advances in Health Economics and Health Services Research*. Greenwich, CN: JAI Press, Inc., forthcoming.

Cohen, Mark A., Eileen J. Tell, and Stanley S. Wallack. "The Lifetime Risks and Costs of Nursing Home Use Among the Elderly." *Medical Care* 24 (December, 1986): 1161–1172.

Employee Benefit Research Institute. "Employer-Sponsored Health Insurance Coverage." *Issue Brief* 58 (September 1986).

————. "Employer-Provided Health Care: Legislative Issues." *Issue Brief* 62 (January 1987).

————. "A Profile of the Nonelderly Population Without Health Insurance." *Issue Brief* 66 (May 1987).

————. "Financing Catastrophic Health Care Costs Among the Nonelderly Population." *Issue Brief* 71 (October 1987).

Friedland, Robert B. "Private Initiatives To Contain Health Care Expenditures." In Frank B. McArdle, ed. *The Changing Health Care Market*. Washington, DC: Employee Benefit Research Institute, 1987.

Fuchs, V.R. "Though Much is Taken: Reflections on Aging, Health, and Medical Care." *Milbank Memorial Fund Quarterly* 62 (Spring 1984):143–166.

Hing, Esther. "Use of Nursing Homes by the Elderly: Preliminary Data From the 1985 National Nursing Home Survey." *NCHS Advancedata* 135 (May 1987).

Howell, Embry; Larry Corder; and Allen Dobson. "Out-of-Pocket Health Expenses for Medicaid Recipients and Low-Income Persons, 1980." In *National Medical Care Utilization and Expenditures Survey*. Series B, Descriptive Report no. 4, DHHS Pub. no. 85-20204. Department of Health and Human Service. Health Care Financing Administration. Office of Research and Demonstrations. Washington, DC: U.S. Government Printing Office, 1985.

Huang, Lien-Fu; Teh-wei Hu; and William S. Cartwright. "The Economic Cost of Senile Dementia in the United States, 1983." Unpublished paper from the U.S. Department of Health and Human

Services, Public Health Service, National Institutes of Health, National Institute on Aging.

Levit, Katherine R.; Helen Lazenby; Daniel R. Waldo; and Lawrence M. Davidoff. "National Health Expenditures, 1984." *Health Care Financing Review* 1 (Fall 1985).

Liu, Korbin; Kenneth G. Manton; and Barbara Liu. "Home Care Expenses for the Disabled Elderly." *Health Care Financing Review* 2 (Winter, 1986): 51–58; table 6.

Manton, Kenneth G., and Korbin Liu. "The Future Growth of the Long-Term Care Population: Projections Based on the 1977 National Nursing Home Survey and the 1982 Long-Term Care Survey." Paper prepared for the Third National Leadership Conference on Long-Term Care Issues: *The Future World of Long-Term Care*. Washington, DC., March 7-9, 1984.

McMillan, Alma; Penelope L. Pine; Marian Gornick; and Ronald Prihoda. "Aged Persons Entitled to Both Medicare and Medicaid." *Health Care Financing Review* 4 (Summer 1983): 19–46.

McMillan, Alma, and Marian Gornick. "The Dually Entitled Elderly Medicare and Medicaid Population Living in the Community." *Health Care Financing Review* 2 (Winter 1984): 73–86.

Reinhardt, Uwe. "Medicare Catastrophic Insurance." Statement before U.S. the Senate Committee on the Budget, February 25, 1987.

Rice, Thomas, and Jon Gabel. "Protecting the Elderly Against High Health Care Costs." *Health Affairs* 3 (Fall 1986): 5–21.

Strahan, Genevieve. "Nursing Home Characteristics: Preliminary Data from the 1985 National Nursing Home Survey." *NCHS Advancedata* 131 (March 27, 1987).

Tilly, Jane, and Debbie Bruner. *Medicaid and its Effect on the Elderly*. Washington, DC: American Association of Retired Persons, 1987.

U.S. Congressional Budget Office. "Cost Estimate: H.R. 2470 as Amended by Committee: The Medicare Catastrophic Protection Act of 1987," June 29, 1987.

U.S. Congressional Budget Office. "Cost Estimate: Amendments to H.R. 2470, Relating to Coverage of Outpatient Drugs under Medicare," July 15, 1987.

U.S. Congressional Budget Office. "Cost Estimate: S.1127: the Medicare Catastrophic Loss Prevention Act of 1987," July 2, 1987.

U.S. Department of Commerce. Census Bureau. *Disability, Functional Limitation, and Health Insurance Coverage: 1984/85*. Current Population Reports, Series P-70, no. 8. U.S. Government Printing Office: Washington, DC., 1986.

U.S. General Accounting Office. *Medicare: Comparison of Catastrophic*

Health Insurance Proposals. Briefing Report to the Chairman, Select Committee on Aging, House of Representatives. Washington, DC: U.S. General Accounting Office, 1987.

U.S. Department of Health and Human Services. Health Care Financing Administration. *1987 Annual Report of the Board of Trustees of the Federal Hospital Insurance Trust Fund,* and *1987 Annual Report of the Board of Trustees of the Federal Supplementary Medical Insurance Trust Fund.* Washington, DC: U.S. Government Printing Office, March 30, 1987.

————. Public Health Service. Nation Center for Health Statistics. *Health Statistics on Older Persons, 1986.* Analytical and Epidemiological Studies, Series 3, no. 25. Washington, DC: U.S. Government Printing Office, 1987.

U.S. Department of Labor. Bureau of Labor Statistics. *Employee Benefits in Medium and Large Firms, 1986.* Washington, DC: U.S. Government Printing Office, 1987.

Waldo, Daniel, and Helen Lazenby. "Demographic Characteristics and Health Care Use and Expenditures by the Aged in the United States: 1977-1984." *Health Care Financing Review* 1 (Fall 1984), table 11.

Wyszewianski, Leon. "Financially Catastrophic and High-Cost Cases: Definitions, Distinctions, and Their Implications of Policy Formulation." *Inquiry* 23 (Winter 1986): 382-394.

VIII. Private Insurance Policies for Catastrophic and Long-Term Health Care Coverage

PAPER BY LAURENCE F. LANE

The Viability of Long-Term Care Insurance

The current debate on catastrophic health protection highlights the fact that, as a society, we are confronting significant issues of caring for our frail and disabled. These problems are magnified when one looks at caring for individuals who, because of a chronic physical or mental condition, are in need of long-term in-home or nursing home services.

Increased longevity and the growth in the population as a whole mean that more people have chronic physical illnesses that hinder their capacity to function. At the same time, fiscal pressures have curtailed the ability of public programs to absorb increasing long-term care costs. This adds urgency to the exploration of alternative ways of caring for people with long-term needs and methods of financing those services. The private sector is responding with creative approaches which meet the needs of a portion of individuals who are at risk.

Alternative Financing Approaches

Informed consumers are increasingly conscious of their risk of needing professional long-term care services, and they are encouraging the development of insurance and related products to assist them in planning and paying for nursing home and home care services.

While the political debate continues as to whether long-term care should be a public good, and, therefore financed through government programs, there is a growing recognition that public programs take a long time to develop and often fall short of their pronounced goals. As the report of the HHS Task Force on Long-Term Health Care Policies documented, there has been significant progress made during the past few years in stimulating innovative private market approaches to long-term care financing (U.S. Department of Health and

Human Services, 1987).* An expansion of these private efforts is essential if individuals are to be encouraged to take responsibility for a portion of their long-term care needs.

As table VIII.1 shows, the private market response can be divided into two categories: health policy oriented and economic policy oriented.

The health policy oriented response defines long-term care needs as a biomedical condition. Under this model, risk factors are tied to specific health status. The underlying need for services is viewed within a continuum of medical and social factors. The response is to provide a benefit that supports professional intervention. Health policy oriented responses take two-forms: mechanisms that are purely financing vehicles and mechanisms that combine financing with the delivery of services.

The economic policy oriented response views the risk of long-term care as a financial condition. The overriding risk is the poverty that might come from outliving one's assets and resources, or that might occur following the onset of a chronic disease or disabling condition. This market response can be divided between targeted and untargeted asset accumulation approaches.

Health Policy Oriented Initiatives

The demand for insurance against the risk of personal exposure for the cost of care has significantly increased. In a relatively short period

TABLE VIII.1
Private Market Approaches to Long-Term Care Financing

Health Policy Oriented	Economic Policy Oriented

Financing:
  individual insurance
  group insurance
  long-term disability
	Targeted asset accumulation
	  retirement medical accounts
	  life insurance with rider
	  deferred annuity

Financing and delivery:
  HMOs and SHMOs
  life care community
  preferred provider
	Untargeted asset accumulation
	  pension and 401(k)
	    accumulation
	  home equity conversion
	  life insurance cash values

*Editor's note: see Appendix B for a summary of this report.

120

of time, feasibility issues have been resolved, products have been successfully test-marketed, and widescale marketing initiatives have been launched. During the past several years, a number of major insurers have entered the market with long-term care insurance products.

Individual Policies—The predominate coverage available today on the market is indemnity insurance sold on an individual policy basis. It is estimated that more than 400,000 policyholders are covered by such private long-term care insurance (U.S. Department of Health and Human Services, 1987). This represents a doubling of the market base in less than two years. Forecasts predict a doubling of both products and covered individuals by 1988.

These individual products have four common features:

(1) As indemnity coverage, the benefit is a preset payment specified in the policy normally as a flat rate per diem. Premiums are determined based upon the level of indemnity selected by the policyholder.

(2) Coverage for professional services is for longer than a six-month period, with most policies covering a minimum of three years of indemnity payments for covered services.

(3) Individual underwriting is exercised by the insurer. Applicants are carefully screened in an effort to eliminate high risks.

(4) Utilization criteria do not limit rehabilitation goals and service provisions as does the Medicare program. (Long-term care insurance differs from Medicare supplemental insurance in that the latter is carefully shaped by the insurer to restrict payment to Medicare-approved treatment. Since Medicare pays for only a small share of extended care services, Medicare supplemental insurance has limited application for long-term care.)

The primary approach to marketing individual indemnity coverage is through local agents. The product is sold as a freestanding coverage. A variation of this marketing strategy has been through mass marketing with a group endorsement. For instance, the American Association of Retired Persons, in cooperation with the Prudential Insurance Company, has developed a group endorsed product, but with individual applicant underwriting.

Table VIII.2 summarizes the key issues that should be considered in reviewing these indemnity products.

Group Coverage—True group insurance coverage for long-term care is a recent development. Several insurers have been working with select continuing care retirement centers (CCRCs) to provide community rated, actuarially determined health coverage. For instance, Provident Life, in conjunction with the actuarial consultants of A.

121

TABLE VIII.2
Long-Term Care Insurance Policy Review

It is estimated that nearly 75 different long-term care insurance policies were available in the market as of October 1987. Policies are available through most major insurers, including Aetna Life Insurance, American Republic Insurance, Amex Life Assurance Company (formerly Fireman's Insurance), Banker's Life and Casualty, Continental Casualty Company, John Hancock Insurance, Mutual of Omaha, Mutual of New York (MONY)/ Bnai B'rith Group, Provident Life, Prudential/AARP Group Plan, Travelers Insurance, and a number of Blue Cross/Blue Shield plans.

In reviewing policies, consideration must be given to the following specifics:

Contract information
  (a) What are the conditions of renewability?
  (b) Is there a ceiling on the age for which applications will be accepted?
  (c) What are the underwriting criteria?

Premium information
  (a) How much are the premiums?
  (b) Under what conditions can the premiums be raised?
  (c) Under what conditions are premiums waived?
  (d) Are there restrictions on who pays the premiums?

Coverage information
  (a) What pre-exisiting conditions are excluded from coverage and for how long?
      Does the policy cover Alzheimer's disease and related organic based illness?
  (b) Does the policy require prior hospitalization?
  (c) Is skilled care required to initiate benefit?
  (d) What levels of long-term care are covered?
      Is there home care coverage?
      Is there custodial care coverage?
      Is the benefit reduced for these levels of care?

Policy Benefits
  (a) Is there an elimination period before the policy begins paying?
  (b) What is the length of benefit?
      Is the coverage reduced for home care and/or custodial care?
  (c) Is the policy subordinate to Medicare and/or other insurance?
  (d) What are the maximum and minimum benefits?
  (e) Can the benefits be directly assigned?
  (f) Are there any special coverages provided (e.g., hospice care)?

Foster Higgins, has marketed a CCRC health insurance coverage which combines Medicare supplementary insurance with long-term care nursing home and home care protection. A major development during 1987 was the growing enthusiasm from insurers who express confidence in broadening group coverage.

This movement toward group plan coverage has received a boost from several quarters. The Commission on College Retirement issued a comprehensive report in mid-summer 1986 designing a prototype group product. About the same time, the Health Insurance Association of America completed a survey of its members indicating that several were designing group products. The Travelers Companies announced preparations to market an employee-group long-term care benefit. Aetna has disclosed that it has entered an agreement to underwrite an expense-incurred (with maximum limits) group product for retired Alaska state employees.

Additionally, a number of the Blue Cross plans, working collaboratively, have shared research on group developments. A real sign of the times is that a group of researchers from the Health Policy Center at Brandeis University have formed a long-term care consulting company, Life Plans, to market group actuarial information.

Related to the development of group long-term care products are a series of explorations concerning the integration of such coverage into other health and/or disability coverages. While no examples of such coverage are currently on the market, there appear to be few obstacles to including an umbrella long-term care coverage component, with a separate, large deductible, in an existing major medical policy. Similarly, at least one company that has experience in the disability insurance market is considering a policy supplement which would expand policy benefits to protect against deferred disability, i.e., a prefunded income supplement product which would be triggered by the onset of a long-term disability.

Financing and Delivery Approaches—Health reforms combining financing and delivery are generally viewed as essential if long-term care coverage is to be integrated into a continuum of services. As experts at a conference on the maturing long-term care insurance market concluded, "Managed care systems are desirable for cost savings, risk control, and utilization control" (American Health Care Association, 1987). The HHS Task Force on Long-Term Health Care Policies urged the expansion of case-managed programs.

At the same time, with the exception of several demonstration projects funded primarily through government waivers and the small risk pooling which occurs in life care and continuing care retirement centers, there are few viable managed long-term care systems. Health maintenance organizations (HMOs) have generally restricted coverage, to avoid exposure for long-term nursing home and home care. Even with expanded Medicare risk sharing, most HMOs have avoided long-term care commitments. At least one HMO group, Group Health of Puget Sound, is offering individual long-term care policies, and several others are looking to serve as brokers for such policies. Under such arrangements, the HMO serves as group sponsor for individual policies sold to enrollees. This is viewed as a first step toward broadening coverage to include long-term care services.

Four sites are experimenting with a social health maintenance organization (S/HMO), which strengthens preventive and community support services for persons in need of long-term interventions. The programs now underway in New York City, Minneapolis (MN), Portland (OR) and Long Beach (CA), are designed to provide experience data with which to develop an actuarial basis for underwriting coverage. The S/HMO takes responsibility for bringing the full range of acute and chronic care services into a single system. A capitated payment is determined for the cost of service, and the entity which sponsors the S/HMO is at risk for service costs.

The growth of integrated corporate providers of long-term care services at the regional and national levels meets a prerequisite of developing a preferred provider organization (PPO). Several of these providers are exploring with third-party payers arrangements under which a preferred contract could be established. Experiments of this nature should be launched in the near future.

Economic Policy-Oriented Approaches

Concerns regarding consumer willingness to prefund long-term health care services have stimulated exploration of savings vehicles that could either be used to finance services or to augment retirement income. Such mechanisms would unlock existing resources available to consumers of long-term care services and/or establish a vested asset which, if unused, could be passed to heirs.

Targeted Asset Accumulation—The creation of a tax-favored individual medical account (IMA) is one of the major recommendations of the Department of Health and Human Services report on catastrophic illness (U.S. Department of Health and Human Services, 1986). Under such a proposal, individuals would be encouraged, through favorable taxation provisions, to save specifically for retirement health care expenses. While the Department of Health and Human Services

124

has not transmitted a specific proposal for the Congress to consider, several members of Congress have introduced legislation that would encourage such a program. Colorado has enacted legislation establishing favorable treatment for such savings; the state program is viewed, however, as a minor incentive compared to federal tax deferral.

Two additional targeted asset accumulation vehicles are being discussed. Life insurance underwriters are exploring the actuarial soundness and pricing of an approach that would unlock the face value of life products at the onset of a chronic disability. Under such an approach, the face value would develop an annuity stream which would augment the purchasing power of the consumer. For an additional premium, life policyholders could receive a disability supplement. There may be need for changes in federal tax law for such products to be widely marketed at an affordable premium.

In the absence of major breakthroughs on such life products, there has been a resurgence of marketing to seniors of lump-sum, deferred annuities. Approaches are being made both as a settlement option of life claims and as freestanding savings products. For example, several retirement centers have endorsed deferred annuities that preserve the value of the estate until a later time. Retired couples entering such retirement centers in their early 70s and in good health are encouraged to invest in a lump sum, paid-up annuity which would be activated if the individuals moved into the medical center.

Untargeted Asset Accumulation—Because conscious consumer thinking about retirement health care needs is required to structure a market for both health-oriented and targeted-asset products, considerable exploration is underway in unlocking other income streams which could be used, if needed, for the purchase of long-term care services.

Since 1950, the median income of the elderly has more than doubled, increasing more quickly over the past two decades than the income of the nonelderly population. Half of the elderly between the ages of 65 and 69 are receiving pension assistance, and within the coming decade this income supplement will be available to nearly four out of five elderly persons. Tapping the pension funding stream for long-term care service funding is a controversial topic, but it needs to be explored. The Employee Benefit Research Institute is to be commended for its leadership in research on long-term care. Northwestern National Life Insurance has broken new ground with its LifeScope Program. LifeScope combines a portable pension fund with both preretirement and postretirement financial counseling, with the

125

goal of preserving people's pension income for their older years. Following through with this initiative, Northwestern National Life is supporting several managed long-term care projects to ascertain if the funding stream can be channeled directly to managed care providers (Northwestern National Life Insurance, 1986).

Unlocking the equity within the home is viewed as one potential way to finance long-term care. Nearly three out of four elderly householders own their own home. Two of the approaches being explored for home equity conversion are reverse annuity mortgages (RAMS) and sale-leaseback arrangements (Jacobs and Weissert, 1984). The RAM is a loan against the equity in a home with the proceeds paid to the borrower in monthly installments, usually over a fixed period of time. Upon maturity, the loan must be repaid or renegotiated. In the sale-leaseback arrangement, homeowners sell their homes to an investor. The seller is guaranteed the right of lifetime occupancy. The investor takes over all responsibilities for taxes and maintenance. When the seller dies, the investor takes full possession of the home. Experiments with both programs have attracted limited interest from the elderly.

Many insurance agents are encouraging individuals who are not ready to purchase a specific long-term care policy to purchase life products with cash value, e.g., universal life insurance. Such life products become an asset that could be converted or borrowed from to purchase necessary long-term care services.

Summary

The primary vehicle for private financing of long-term care services currently on the market is an individual indemnity product. Initiatives are underway to broaden the options for the consumer.

Considerable progress has been made during the past few years in stimulating private market exploration of financing long-term care. Perhaps the most significant benchmark to judge progress is the number of insurance companies that are weighing the risks of entering the market against the risk of not entering and missing a market opportunity. At the same time, a realistic market assessment indicates that most insurers are proceeding cautiously.

In the absence of a strong data base, companies are experimenting in product design, marketing, pricing, and control. Sales and market experience continue to generate additional data that are being used to revise market approaches. Moreover, insurers are going beyond traditional product lines. Hybrid experimentation combining features of health, life, disability, and pension products are being tested.

At this stage of market development, there is optimism that the innovation, creativity, and risk taking needed to overcome market development barriers will be applied.

The issue of how to finance long-term care is not going to go away. As public attention to it increases, the debate about who should shoulder what part of the costs—individual consumers; federal, state, or local governments; and/or private employers—will certainly intensify. As more individuals and families experience firsthand the inadequacies of the current system, collective pressures to respond will be exerted on both the private and public sectors. If the response to long-term care follows the course of responses to other domestic needs, it will result in a patchwork of options tailored to meet differing consumer needs. The private insurance market will continue as one of those options.

References

American Health Care Association. Private Long-Term Care Insurance: The Maturing Market. Conference Summary. San Antonio, Texas, January 13–14, 1987.

Commission on College Retirement. *A Plan to Create Comprehensive Group Long Term Care Insurance for College and University Personnel.* New York, NY: Commission on College Retirement, July 1986.

Health Insurance Association of America. "The State of Private Long Term Care Insurance: Results from a National Survey." *Research and Statistical Bulletin* 5 (November 1986).

Jacobs Paul, and William Weissert. *Home Equity Financing of Long Term Care for the Elderly.* Chapel Hill, NC: University of North Carolina, January 1984 (reprint).

Northwestern National Life Insurance. *America's Health Care Challenge: New Directions for Business, Government and Individuals.* Symposium report, January 27, 1986.

U.S. Department of Health and Human Services. Health Care Financing Administration. *Report of the Task Force on Long Term Health Care Policies.* Washington, DC: U.S. Government Printing Office, 1987.

————. *Catastrophic Illness Expenses: A Report to the President.* Washington, DC: U.S. Government Printing Office, 1986.

IX. How Do We Begin?

REMARKS OF JANET MYDER

The Need for Coverage

MS. MYDER: In reviewing the issues related to assessing the need for catastrophic and long-term health care coverage, I surveyed a wide range of concerns. These included defining what are catastrophic health care costs and asking, what do we really want to protect ourselves against?

I think we have covered the definitions quite well. In order to assess the need for coverage or examine the coverage that currently exists, whether public or private, we need to define "catastrophic." We have been told that examining personal expenditures or financial liability is a starting point. Levels of out-of-pocket expenditures, individual and family incomes, and current public or private insurance coverage all need to be figured into the definition. Thus we can determine what is catastrophic to specific population groups and then measure the need for additional or improved third party coverage.

We understand that the catastrophic needs of younger people are medical needs. The catastrophic needs of the over-65 population are long-term care needs. I would stress—and this has been clearly pointed out—that when we are talking about the younger population, we may also be talking about long-term care needs.

The nursing home industry is caring for increasing numbers of younger people. While technology is helping older people live longer, it is also helping younger people live longer after traumatic injuries, and these people need care for many years. As John Rother pointed out in reference to the elderly, the need for long-term care covers a more extended period of time than the need for medical care. However, older people also incur catastrophic *medical* expenditures. In part, those expenditures are addressed by the Medicare Catastrophic Coverage Act of 1988. Others, such as the balance billing for physicians' care under Medicare Part B, are not covered.

In identifying coverage needs, Robert Friedland mentioned that having insurance, whether it is public or private, does not necessarily mean having sufficient protection. The presence or absence of insurance is a measure of coverage, but identifying the uninsured can be accomplished by viewing adequacy of coverage relative to specific services for which people are at risk.

For example, of the 20 to 40 million people under the age of 65 who have no insurance or are underinsured, almost any episode of acute illness or injury can be catastrophic. By the same token, there are 28 million older people who are essentially uninsured for long-term care expenditures. These are people who have Medicare coverage and supplemental Medigap coverage. However, they are uninsured for long-term care.

When we look at out-of-pocket expenses that do not include the cost of nursing home care and the cost of community-based long-term care services, we see that older people are reasonably well covered for medical expenses. Adding long-term care expenses into the equation, however, demonstrates how woefully inadequate is that coverage.

For example, as Robert Friedland pointed out, in 1984, $32 billion was spent on nursing home care for older people. Medicare covered only 1.9 percent of its cost and private insurance barely 1 percent. Out-of-pocket payments covered 49 percent and Medicaid 43 percent.

The Potential of Financing Alternatives

How do we begin, or, where do we begin?

I would like to mention the AARP-Villers poll because it provides us with a good reference point. Even though the people surveyed were not given a choice of options between "leaving long-term care entirely to the individual" or "considering some kind of government action or program," the messages from that survey are very important. Average citizens who answered those questions are probably further along than public policymakers and possibly many of us in answering these questions.

These are the people who deal day-to-day with the long-term care system as it currently exists. They are the informal caregivers. They have to sacrifice some family relationships to take care of elders in the home or out of the home. They also have to miss work or cut back on their employment in order to be informal caregivers.

The key to the survey results is that the general public seems to know that we have to spend money—whether public or private—to take care of the nation's long-term care needs, and we have to act soon.

The question arises, what are we doing? What measures are underway? Laurence Lane clearly pointed out that there is some promise in private insurance. We have a long way to go, but I think we are off to a good start.

We need to remind ourselves that the 450,000 policies currently in force represent coverage for only 1.5 percent of the over-65 population. If we triple the number of policies in force, that will cover barely 5 percent of today's elderly.

Optimism about Private Insurance

If we look more closely at the kind of coverage available, there are reasons for us to be optimistic about private insurance. It is expected to cover a significant part, though only a part, of total long-term care needs.

Insurers are considering long-term care in a broader sense now. They are looking at health care, disability coverage, and retirement income and encouraging innovation in the administration of benefits. They are also looking at managed care and proposals to base benefits on functional levels rather than on the need for specific services, to redefine the group, and to integrate long-term care with other existing benefits. These are directions that the market needs to take for private insurance to make a significant impact on part of the long-term care financing requirement.

Another question is how to stimulate further development. All of us should recognize that a public program alone is not going to be the answer, nor is a private program.

Some combination of public and private financing will help to cover today's older population and prepare for the future. Bringing younger workers into the insurance pools will ultimately lead to a comprehensive long-term care system that meets the needs of virtually all of the population.

What Do We Want to Protect?

A final comment. What do we want to protect?

What do we risk losing when there is no long-term care coverage, whether public, private, or some combination? Some obvious answers are assets, income, and savings. The financial security of spouses and their eventual long-term care protection are also at risk.

We risk losing choices. These include the ability of people who have a need for long-term care to choose the nature or the site of services that they receive and to choose how they spend the last years of their lives. We may also risk the opportunity to preserve family relations.

Inter-generational harmony is at risk when caregivers, mostly women, must leave work to care for the elderly. We need to protect productivity also. Finally, individual dignity and, ultimately, the dignity of society as a whole, will be protected if we take care of the population's long-term care needs.

These are important questions to address and important areas to preserve as we proceed with defining and designing a comprehensive long-term care financing plan.

X. Part Three Discussion

A Vision of What Is Needed

MR. LEONARD: I am reminded of a quote that was used at a recent conference: "If you don't know where you're going, any road will get you there." What has been lacking in the long-term care debate is a vision. What is it that we want? We have been talking about the mechanics of long-term care—whether public or private—who is going to pay for it, how it should be defined. But, really, we should be talking about strategic planning. Again, what is our vision?

Is there a single, comprehensive, agreed upon, benchmark vision that makes sense? For example, is it the recognition of personal dignity, of being able to live out one's life in an acceptable manner? Is it that the government has a responsibility to take care of people?

MR. JACKSON: We have been consulting with a number of clients on long-term care coverage, and while each one has a specific set of problems, I think they share a common goal.

In our own case (The Wyatt Company), one year ago we considered a long-term disability plan. After lengthy discussion, we finally concluded we could not adopt it, but cost was not the problem.

We could fit the cost in prospectively. We could fund this coverage by giving it priority over other needs. Basically, we could not adopt the plan because we didn't feel it was responsible to promise something that we could not arrange to finance. In short, we could not fund it.

Long-term care is like a pension, in effect. Many people will be reaching retirement. Perhaps one out of four or one out of five will face catastrophic illness. We could very easily design coverage as part of the pension vehicle, but you cannot fund long-term care, and so we just gave up on that mechanism.

We have a case in one of our major offices of a secretary who retired after 10 years of service and is now in a nursing home. She has one son who earns, I think, $11,000 a year and is married and cannot afford long-term care expenses, and her profit-sharing fund will run out soon. Our basic approach is that we will take care of one of our retirees one way or another. We will do it on an ad hoc out-of-pocket basis because there is no formal mechanism available. So, we are aware of the need.

I think many companies would be prepared to do something, but they are faced with a huge obligation for benefits they have already promised to retirees that they cannot fund. Taking on yet another obligation would seem to be irresponsible.

So, we have opted, basically, for our own form of private charity.

Gatekeeping Mechanisms

MS. SCHAEFFER: No insurance policy that I know of claims to cover all nursing needs, whether the care is in a nursing home or in a residence. We are all trying to exclude what we would call unnecesssary uses, or in some cases, abuses. Otherwise costs would escalate and, in the end, the policy would not be insurance.

Every insurance company has tried to come up with some sort of gatekeeping mechanism to separate the "necessaries" from the "unnecessaries."

You have seen these gatekeepers in the form of requirements for three-days of hospitalization, in higher levels of nursing care need before lower levels, and in the functional necessity. However, I would assert that the result of these requirements is to exclude some quite legitimate needs for nursing. So I do not think any of us have yet solved the question of how to design insurance to cover real needs. Furthermore, I do not think the solution can necessarily be found in the private sector or in the public sector.

What people are looking for is comprehensive coverage at a minimal price, and it is not there.

Defining the Insurable Event

MR. LANE: I would like to emphasize that there has been a lot of searching for a definition of the "insurable event." What is the promise that we are willing to make?

At the heart of my comments is a sense of a frustrated public response to the issue. At this stage of long-term care development, we are not at a point where we can come up with a comprehensive solution. If we are going to make any progress at all, it will be by small steps. Those small steps will involve different definitions of what the insurable event should be, but the definition will generally take into consideration: (1) the population being insured; (2) whatever that group relationship is; (3), the service market area; and (4) experimental approaches to managing that service structure.

I never realized the fragility of the long-term care system until I was on the vendor-supplier side, selling a service. I am beginning to realize the weakness of the administrative structure at the point of service delivery. This system is overtaxed even in terms of meeting its basic priority—nursing—and yet we expect it to do much more.

Small steps are the best we can hope for at this stage. A multiple set of building blocks will help us determine what the vision should be.

The Role of Medicaid in Providing Long-Term Care Services

MR. VLADECK: I question Laurence Lane's description of the "Medicaid mentality," or the impossibility of giving any kind of adequate care under Medicaid.

I am not a former Medicaid director, but I used to set Medicaid nursing home rates. While I would not begin to try to defend the basic dynamics of Medicaid eligibility, or other aspects of Medicaid, the program has done an extremely good job of providing long-term care services for those who become recipients of this benefit.

In every community that I know of, elderly persons, in a hospital or in the community, who need long-term care services, are much better off if they have Medicaid coverage than if they do not and cannot afford the out-of-pocket expense of care.

There have never been any data to demonstrate that facilities with higher proportions of private paying patients provide better care than facilities with mostly Medicaid patients. There is a great deal of variation from one community to another that does not correlate at all with the extent of Medicaid coverage.

Most facilities that have many private-pay patients—with the exception of maybe 2 to 3 percent of all facilities—have Medicaid patients in the same facilities. In fact, most Medicaid patients used to be private patients in those facilities. I do not believe that the nursing homes reduce the level of service for those folks once they go on Medicaid, at least not in most states. If they do, they do so illegally.

Medicaid is cheap. It is cheap in terms of retention, of total expense in relation to what is paid out to providers. It provides low-cost long-term care with only indirect restrictions on freedom of choice.

Historically, I think it is correct to say that the initial impetus for long-term care insurance in the private sector came from providers who knew that, by definition, any private insurance system would pay them more per unit of service than Medicaid would pay. I suggest that has some lessons for those of you who are getting into the business of writing private insurance.

If you start stigmatizing Medicaid because it is welfare and, therefore, by definition, it is inadequate in this society, you miss a lot of what is actually happening in long-term care. You can go down some very misleading paths in terms of how the long-term care system is likely to evolve or should evolve.

To the extent that in some communities an infrastructure is beginning to develop for the delivery of relatively coherent, relatively well-organized long-term care, it is Medicaid that is doing that organizing.

Use of Medicaid by the Middle Class

MR. PRESS: I am an ex-Medicaid director. A major concern of mine when I was a Medicaid director in Connecticut was equity in the program.

My concern was the extensive use of Medicaid's long-term care program by the middle class, and the strains that it put on the program in terms of reducing benefits for the poor. I have not heard much about that today, but as an ex-Medicaid director who was also at the American Health Care Association, I viewed long-term care insurance in a very positive way. It was strongly supported by those in the government and other Medicaid directors because it was looked upon as an opportunity to reduce the cost of supporting long-term care for the middle class.

It was also looked upon as giving the middle class an opportunity to provide for its own needs, which is positive. Some of this is in response to Bruce Vladeck's comment about the equality of treatment between private and nonprivate patients in nursing homes.

If there is a mix of private and nonprivate patients in an individual nursing home, it is likely that there will be no discrimination and that the care will be equal. But anyone who has compared the care in a 100-percent private-pay facility with that in a 100-percent Medicaid facility must realize that when the Medicaid facility only costs $35 or $40 a day for room, board, and health care in a number of states, the care cannot be the same as that given in the average private-pay facility, which charges twice that amount. I think we also have to provide the opportunity for the middle class to use private facilities. It would be a positive opportunity for them as well as for the government. If middle-class people continue to transfer their assets to their children, which was the practice that I encountered in my Medicaid years and that still exists today, they are feeding into that second tier of the system, the lower tier, and lesser care. I am not sure that many people are completely aware of what it means when they move their money to trusts, etc.; but, essentially, they are setting themselves up for lesser care.

So, providing the middle class with an opportunity to provide for itself is positive for them, and I think it is positive for the government. It may be positive for the poor, as well, in terms of an effort to push private long-term insurance.

Ms. YOUNG: There are always people who say that what is wrong with farm programs in this country is that the people who write them do not understand how smart farmers are, and I think this is the same situation.

The middle class has been given an opportunity by attorneys to shelter some of their wealth and let Medicaid (which they note they have paid for in taxes all these years) take care of them if they need long-term care. If you try to design a two-tier program that has the middle class pay through purchases of insurance, with the poor being paid for through a public program, then you may put yourself in the same situation. Unlike other benefits that were designed that way, this benefit shows no signs of being paid for by employers.

So, in essence, you are going to be saying to the middle class, "Pay for it yourself, and then your taxes will pay for those who don't elect to pay for it." I wonder whether anybody has thought about the questions in that message.

If you are going to design a two-tier program, you must design it so there is some reason why workers should take that money out of current earnings to provide for themselves in the future.

Nursing Home Length of Stay

MR. SALISBURY: Is it not arguable that one reason is simply that it would spare a person from having to face the spending-down of all of his or her assets since, as the statistics indicate, many people who go into nursing homes are not going there for the remainder of their lives but only for a period?

Ms. YOUNG: Much of that period *is* the remainder of life, I think, because it is not acute care that we are talking about.

MR. LANE: Both the National Nursing Home Survey in 1977 and the recent 1985 edition show that about a third of the individuals who enter the nursing home setting are discharged within the first three months of entry.

Ms. YOUNG: And those are acute-care patients?

137

MR. LANE: Do not get confused with acute care. They are generally restorative, or recouperative, or have a condition that allows them to be discharged.

MS. YOUNG: And Medicare pays for their care.

MR. LANE: They may be Medicare eligible but most likely they are not. That is because the length-of-stay payment under Medicare is very truncated, about 20 days, for those who qualify for a skilled nursing facility (SNF).*

About 40 percent or so of the nursing home population remains in the nursing home for longer than two years, and that portion has been growing. This aging-in-place syndrome often is related to Alzheimer's disease or to incontinence and multiple limitations in the activities of daily living.

The remaining percentages represent individuals whose condition is usually terminal and who are often discharged from the nursing home setting to another component of the health care system, such as a hospital environment. This is the group for whom death is a near certainty.

Let us at least begin to clarify what we are talking about before we design the ultimate system. We still have a tendency to speak of nursing homes as a single instrument. Nursing homes serve at least three different populations, often within the same facility, because of failures in existing public policy.

MS. YOUNG: But it seems to me that if Congress had to legislate the sharing of pensions because many workers were not opting for spousal coverage, many workers today may not be concerned about whether their spouses would become impoverished if they had to go into a nursing home in their old age. That is what we are facing. In designing a program, there would be a real need to help workers understand why they should pay out of their own pocket for insurance coverage.

Workers Willing to Pay for Coverage

MR. SALISBURY: The evidence from the surveys that have been noted is that a large percentage of workers say they would be willing to pay for some level of coverage and would want to buy some protection. Whether that is a sufficient number or just gets us to the 30

---

*Editor's note: Under the Medicare Catastrophic Coverage Act of 1988, 150 days of skilled nursing services will be covered starting in 1989.

percent figure that John Rother used as a reasonable success ratio in the view of the informed, or some other number, is an open question.

Ms. YOUNG: What do you do if you design a two-tier program and those who do not participate are left without a means of being taken care of?

MR. SALISBURY: After they have totally spent down, they move into the Medicaid program.

Ms. YOUNG: Wouldn't that appear intelligent to a lot of people?

MR. SALISBURY: This is purely anecdotal, but I know that there are a fair number of people who fall into the category of the American Express program in which active workers are willing to pay for the long-term care insurance for their mothers and fathers to ensure that their parents do not have to spend away the little inheritance the individual might otherwise get.

You may be understating, to some degree, the desire to preserve assets among those with the ability to pay—obviously, only those with an ability to pay. The willing, voluntary purchase of life insurance by such large numbers of Americans, I would argue, supports the argument that many people will be willing to purchase long-term-care insurance.

MR. JACKSON: First of all, practically every major program that is operating successfully today—such as group life insurance, hospital, medical, surgical, major medical, long-term disability—started out on an employee-pay-all basis or an employee-pay-most basis. Gradually they have shifted to the point where the company now pays it all. So, starting out on an employee-pay-all basis does not necessarily mean that that is where you end up.

The second point concerns demographics—what happens in the year 2040 when there will be four retirees for every active worker, and one of the four retirees is in a nursing home. What this implies is that this country may end up with something on the order of 15 to 20 percent of the labor force working in nursing homes. The problem may get beyond financing questions. Other solutions might well be discussed.

What Is the State's Role?

Ms. FELICE: I would like to discuss some of Laurence Lane's questions with him. One concerns whether private insurers are responding

139

to the market and the other was whether the government's role should be to facilitate.

I think Mr. Lane answered "yes" in both cases, but in Massachusetts we have been in a process of finding ways to involve private insurance in the market. We discussed this idea with a large number of people over the last two years, and have come to the conclusion that private insurance would come in the market. To the question of whether that private insurance would participate in a way that solves the social dilemma for elders and for the Medicaid budget, however, our answer was: "Not without a lot of pushing from us."

Should our role then be to facilitate any kind of private insurance activity in the market, or should we act as an initiator of a program that needs to be developed. I think that has been our bias.

I think that the idea of taking small steps forward in this area, as though we lack information about long-term care, is a great misunderstanding. The state carries much of the expense and responsibility for long-term care, and we know a great deal about the people who need it because we deny it on a regular basis until they are income-eligible.

We have had a lot of experience in defining eligibility. It is scary to think about having a private insurer take the risk for that. But given that the state pays for such a great share already and has *all* of the risk, we have a very strong incentive to create, demand, or encourage the kind of private insurance development that will offer a broad spectrum of care, rather than leave many people uncovered.

We have been considering ways of asking people to pay according to their ability to pay. I am not as discouraged as some are about the possibility of means testing, especially for a new benefit. We went backward and tried to means test Medicare after it had already been an acknowledged benefit, but I think our population is generally willing to pay for a new benefit. It just makes a more difficult administrative task for us to design a method of doing it.

MR. LIFSON: Private-sector activity will not increase in this area in order to save state budgets; that is not the reason private-sector activity occurs. It might be one of the benefits of increased private sector activity, but it will not be the reason why companies will risk their own capital it in this area.

If the state wishes to encourage some activity, it has to recognize why companies enter markets and how they organize themselves to respond to what *they* perceive as the demand, which is not necessarily what others define as demand. In the Deficit Reduction Act of 1984, the U.S. Congress inadvertently took away any reasonable way for an employer to participate in this area on a reasonable financial basis. I don't know if it was a lack of vision or a lack of funds. Congress said that the funds were not available to do it. There is a concern that someone will actually respond to this problem and spend too much money—I am not sure it is real money—and yet some members of Congress are advocating increased public programs. So, I have trouble reconciling these two—on the one hand, Congress saying "We cannot have people respond to this rather soft incentive that was in DEFRA because that is going to cost too much federal revenue" and, on the other hand, demand for increased public activity without the ability to finance it.

Public Awareness

Ms. EIN LEWIN: One reason often cited in assessing why the private market has not had broader appeal is that people perceive that they are well covered for long-term care under existing programs such as Medicare and Medicaid. AARP has done some polls to support this contention.

I hear that now that we are getting a different message, there is increasing awareness that long-term care benefits are not adequately provided under existing programs. What impact has this new awareness had on the private market for long-term care insurance?

MR. ROTHER: The AARP-Villers Foundation poll definitely shows the impact of public awareness on the catastrophic care debate that we have been having in public over the last year. Awareness is still poor, but it is much better than it was before.

In terms of the number of people who could correctly assess how much long-term care coverage they have under Medicare, probably about 60 percent of the total population today understands roughly what is covered and what is not. Before the catastrophic coverage debate, a great majority mistakenly believed that they had coverage.

So, we still have a problem with 40 percent of the population, but that is perhaps only half the problem we had two years ago.

MR. FRIEDLAND: A question was raised concerning our goals or our vision concerning the subject of this conference. I would like to offer my sense of what that vision is. We are discussing financing—but, in many ways, this is a means to an end. In the end, we are concerned about the delivery of health care in an efficient and effective manner; about removing the barriers that exist between different kinds of long-term care and those that exist between long-term care and other forms of care, and about establishing a continuum of care. The simple problem of trying to get a physician to go to a nursing home is an example. In pursuing this end we will develop an understanding of how long-term care should be delivered. I do not think we have a full sense, for example, of what a nursing home should look like. What is the most efficient and most effective way of delivering this sort of care?

MR. LANE: I just wanted to respond to Ms. Felice by saying that I think the state is the appropriate level to do planning, and, if a state desires, to reconfigure its current service expenditure in a way that could facilitate a significant system change.

I do not believe that it is an either/or issue. Janet Myder was correct when she said we are talking about a little bit of both. The objective of the private sector insurer may not be the same as that of the public sector, particularly in terms of universality. The goal of the private sector is fairness, that is, treating its policyholders in a fair and equitable way to secure the covered service.

I think you are correct in saying the state should be able to define its role. The state may want to look at how it can reconfigure its expenditures. The federal government should not prevent the state from looking at that. For instance, I have suggested that when a state looks at disabled people whom it currently insures under the SSI (Supplemental Security Income) program, that the state should know for sure that it will have an expenditure for health care needs for them in future years.

Unfortunately, the budget process does not allow for the development of an actuarily sound insurance system that includes an ability to prepay or design a prepayment system for the targeted population. I think that states should have that opportunity. I believe we should look at the tax issues involved in encouraging individuals and insurers to use existing vehicles in a tax-favorable way. This is one of the key recommendations of the Task Force on Long-Term Health Care Policies.*

The task force recommendations dealing with the tax issues call for a policy which would bring long-term care coverage more into line with practices associated with life insurance structures rather than the design currently used in health care. It is not an either/or. When we suggest that a federalized public sector initiative is the solution, we begin to turn debate away from a discussion of the in-

---

*Editor's note: see Appendix B.

cremental steps that can be taken—steps which could encourage states as well as insurers and individuals to begin to act. I do not want to limit the debate on solutions by adopting an either/or position when what is needed is a combination.

PART FOUR
PUBLIC AND PRIVATE ROLES IN CATASTROPHIC AND LONG-TERM CARE

Part Four examines the question of who should assume responsibility for financing catastrophic and long-term care expenses: individuals, families, employers, health service providers, or government.

F. Peter Libassi argues that everyone in society ultimately pays—through taxes, premiums, higher prices on goods and services, and tradeoffs in public programs (chapter XI). He argues that the *real* question is how the price can be paid in a manner that optimizes value.

The current system produces unacceptable consequences, Libassi says, which result from the distribution of the burden among those who pay for care and from the structure of the reimbursement programs. As an example, he cites the large number of middle-class persons who have been forced onto Medicaid after exhausting their savings and assets, although the program is intended for needy persons. This situation not only impoverishes many middle-class persons and their dependents, he adds, but also makes it more difficult for the poor to qualify for Medicaid. While the Medicare Catastrophic Coverage Act of 1988 affords some protection to spouses of institutionalized recipients, Libassi notes, it makes only a small improvement in the protection of long-term care costs.

Federal lawmakers are not willing, however, to make major program expansions to cover long-term care, Libassi says, in view of the federal deficit and cost containment. Employers also face disincentives to participating in the financing of long-term care, such as tax policies and increasing pressures for cost containment.

The answer, Libassi believes, lies in integrated and complementary programs of public and private financing. He describes the recommendations of the Connecticut Commission on Private and Public Responsibilities for Financing Long Term Care for the Elderly. The commission calls for an increase in the variety and availability of new methods of private long-term care financing, expansion of community-based alternatives to institutional care, development of long-range strategies and consumer education programs, and improvement of data collection efforts and public dissemination of information.

What is the role of employers? In chapter XII, Thomas O'Brien and Richard Woodbury discuss the need for colleges and universities to address the issues of inflation and long-term disability, which affect their retirees. Using Harvard University as an example, the authors examine the issues confronting universities, such as the difference between the forms of compensation that employees want and the forms they need.

O'Brien and Woodbury describe the benefit programs at Harvard which, while extensive, do not include coverage for long-term care. Harvard is, however, evaluating the possibility of offering a long-term care insurance plan in partnership with an insurance company. Such a program raises the issue of tradeoffs, such as younger employees subsidizing older workers and retirees and healthy employees subsidizing the disabled retirees.

The authors explore the question of why employers would consider long-term care insurance, given the high cost, the politically unpopular tradeoffs, and the uncertainties surrounding the issue. They conclude that if employers are concerned about income security for their employees in retirement, then some sort of employer-sponsored long-term care insurance is essential.

John J. McCormack contends in chapter XIII that it is only a question of how and when employer-sponsored long-term care plans will be available, not *whether* it will happen. The reason: government mandates in recent years that have expanded employer responsibilities for benefit programs.*

McCormack sees several advantages to providing long-term care through employer-sponsored programs. The cost of insurance is lower through group plans; payroll deduction is more acceptable than out-of-pocket payments; and the benefit can be offered as an add-on to an existing medical plan, he says. Despite these advantages, McCormack maintains, employer plans are not widely available because of cost and because until recently few long-term care products have been available from insurance companies.

McCormack describes the barriers both employers and insurers must overcome if they are to offer long-term care benefits. He then reviews efforts by employers such as the state of Alaska and the Travelers Corporation and by insurers such as the Teachers Insurance and Annuity Association to provide a long-term care benefit.

---

*Editor's note: For further information, see Employee Benefit Research Institute, *Government Mandating of Employee Benefits*, Washington, D.C.: Employee Benefit Research Institute, 1987.

In chapter XIV, Robert M. Ball argues that catastrophic acute-care coverage should be added to basic insurance protection for current workers as well as to Medicare. While the Catastrophic Coverage Act of 1988 provides older persons with protection for acute care, the next major step for this older population group is federal coverage for long-term care, he says.

After discussing the possibilities and problems of insurance and individual savings to meet the cost of long-term care, Ball considers a partnership between a federal insurance program and private insurance. He concludes that the role of a basic government plan would be to provide coverage without a significant waiting period, and the role of private insurance would be to sell supplementary protection to those who could afford it and who wanted additional services or wanted to protect assets.

Ball describes what he sees as the advantages of a social insurance plan and how he believes costs could be contained under such a plan. Finally, he answers the question: "Why social insurance instead of a means-tested program based on Medicaid principles?" People more readily accept a program where eligibility for benefits grows out of past earnings or contributions without a test of need for benefits, he concludes.

In chapter XV, Karen Ignagni says that the Pension Benefit Guaranty Corporation, the federal agency that insures the defined benefit pension promises made to employees, might offer a model for dealing with the long-term care problem because of its limited reinsurance function. Long-term care is not just a health issue, she says, but should be viewed as pension systems are—with an eye to the long term.

Employers face difficult problems and challenges if they try to take on the problem themselves, she says. There are no economies of scale or efficiencies in a system in which employers each try to develop different types of benefits. Ignagni believes that problems of competition could arise if one company offers the benefit and another has lower labor costs because it does not.

Ignagni also comments on the lack of interest shown by young workers—both white- and blue-collar—in this issue, which seems far removed from their lives.

In the Part Four Discussion that follows in chapter XVI, forum participants suggest that public-private partnerships at the state level could provide leadership in the provision of long-term care insurance products and mention the possible role of the federal government in providing tax incentives to encourage private sector initiatives.

XI. Whose Responsibility Is It?

PAPER BY F. PETER LIBASSI

The issue of "responsibility" in financing health and long-term care expenses gives rise to both public policy and ethical questions. This is clear in the examination of even a trite example: an 85-year-old woman with a 50-year history of smoking, poor nutrition, lack of exercise, and other self-abusive lifestyle habits, which she knew would compromise her well-being, becomes ill with chronic lung disease, peripheral circulatory disorders, and osteoporosis. She obviously needs medical and supportive care, but she has no insurance coverage and does not (yet) qualify for Medicaid. She can afford to pay out of pocket for some, but not all, of the needed services. Should this individual pay the consequences of her own lifestyle? Should her children pay for her care or care for her out of a sense of family responsibility? Should her past employer pay for her service needs since it provides other forms of retirement security? Should physicians, hospitals, and nursing homes deliver her care regardless of payment because they have taken the Hippocratic oath or because they are in the business of caring for people? Should the tobacco manufacturers pay for her care because smoking compromised her health? Should the state and/ or federal government step in to provide for her because it is government's role to look after the well-being of its citizens—regardless of their income and economic status? Should society (people of means), through taxes or insurance premiums, pay for her care in the spirit of common cause or economic efficiency?

This simple example illustrates that multiple parties can be held responsible and that the issue can reasonably be addressed only by recognizing that we all are, and will continue to be, responsible for the catastrophic health and long-term costs incurred by members of our society, including the elderly.

Given that we all ultimately pay—through taxes, premiums, higher prices for goods and services, direct caregiving activities, trade-offs in public programs, and emotional energy—the real questions are How can the price we already pay be paid in a manner that optimizes value? How can current financing methods be made more rational, equitable, affordable, predictable, and humane? And what role can and should each responsible party play in that financing system?

To examine these questions, we must first acknowledge the unacceptable consequences of the current system. Second, we must be realistic about the actual potential for implementing new financing arrangements in the current fiscal and political environment. Last, we must draw conclusions and make recommendations about the future of financing catastrophic and long-term care, the latter really being the most common catastrophic health care expense facing the elderly. In view of Congress' activity on catastrophic benefit additions to Medicare, the focus of this paper is on long-term care.

The Current System

As already described, national expenditures for long-term care (more than $32 billion in 1984) are paid for in roughly equal shares by the government (state and federal)—primarily through Medicaid—and by personal, out-of-pocket payments. Medicare, the Veteran's Administration, the Older Americans Act, the Social Services Block Grant, and private insurance also contribute small amounts, which, taken together, pay less than 10 percent of the bill nationwide.

One important source not always recognized in the current financing equation is informal, unpaid care. It is estimated that 80 percent of all long-term care is delivered "free" by family and friends. As we debate proposals to modify the current financing system, we all must exercise care to consider the response and reaction of this informal service delivery system to the introduction of new incentives and disincentives.

The negative aspects of our current system derive less from the relative contributions of each source than from the distribution of the burden within each payer class and from the structure of the reimbursement programs. Attempts to compensate or control for the system's current shortcomings seem to beget additional shortcomings.

Medicaid funds are appropriately directed at supporting the needs of persons unable to finance their own care. However, the means-testing requirements of the program have led many middle-class persons to "spend down" their savings and assets. The means testing requirement of the program has resulted in the impoverishment not only of many individuals but more tragically, their dependents and spouses. Furthermore, these assets and income eligibility requirements provide perverse incentives for persons to protect their life savings by divesting of them in order to establish financial eligibility for Medicaid.

The growing portion of formerly nonpoor elderly on the Medicaid rolls has geometrically increased Medicaid expenditures, straining already-stretched state resources. As state Medicaid programs have

150

tightened eligibility requirements to compensate for increasing per capita outlays, the percentage of those below the poverty level receiving Medicaid assistance dropped from 65 percent in 1976 to 38 percent in 1983. The resulting diminished access to care for many poor, who are unable to qualify for Medicaid, increases pressure on states to find alternative long-term care financing sources and to contain costs. Many states have done so by underpaying service providers. The widening differentials between private rates and Medicaid reimbursement rates discourage service providers from accepting Medicaid patients. Access to both institutional and community-based care is often thereby limited. Access to noninstitutional alternatives is also limited in many states because community-based services are not covered through Medicaid. Funds may be available for these services through other public programs. However, navigating the fragmented systems of both financing and delivering long-term care services is a complex task for a well person and may be quite overwhelming to an elderly individual compromised by crisis and functional disability.

All of these objectionable aspects of the current system translate to a human cost: older Americans needing long-term care services feel stripped of independence, dignity, and control over their own lives. The current long-term care financing system leads people either to impoverishment or to gaming the system by transferring assets. It results in inappropriate institutionalization and is irrational, inequitable, and inadequate. This system came about by default, not by design.

The challenge is to design a comprehensive, coordinated system that will moderate the growth in public expenditures for long-term care, assist families to meet their long-term care financial needs, and assist families to find the care services needed by the elderly and their families.

The Environment for Reform

Looking at long-term care solely as a financing issue, no single sector of society or the economy appears able or willing to take on the entire burden, or even to assume major added responsibility, to relieve others of their current financing burden.

The Medicare Catastrophic Coverage Act of 1988 makes a laudable first step by expanding coverage for pharmaceuticals, skilled nursing care, and home health care and by affording some protection from impoverishment to community-residing spouses of institutionalized

151

Medicaid recipients. However, this legislation represents only a small improvement in protection for most Medicare beneficiaries who already have private insurance but still have no protection from the most frequent cause of catastrophic health care expense—long-term care. The message from Congress is clear—lawmakers are not willing to make major program expansions to cover long-term care.

Furthermore, an enlarged federal government program would not be likely to provide the level of choice and variety consumers want, the sensitivity to local needs and resources that is necessary, or the adaptability to changing demands and technologies that are inevitable in this rapidly evolving field.

In any event, congressional and administration attention are focused on the federal deficit and cost containment, limiting the likelihood of any major expansion of the federal role in long-term care.

State governments are also searching for ways to contain, not expand, their responsibilities for long-term care expenses. In Connecticut, Medicaid expenditures for nursing home care rose 255 percent in 10 years, from $77.1 million in 1977 to a budgeted $273.7 million in 1987. In the same period the overall state budget only grew 174 percent. With no moderation in the rate of long-term care spending under Medicaid, these state nursing home expenditures could consume as much as 7.9 percent of the budget by the year 2000. Other states, especially those with less healthy economies, are experiencing even worse fiscal crises as they seek to stem their growing long-term care expenditures through measures ranging from tougher Medicaid means tests, to moratoria on nursing home bed construction, to the financing of lower cost care alternatives under waiver experiments. In the future, however, state Medicaid programs will remain a key source for funding long-term care services.

In the private sector, employers—the major vehicle for distribution of health insurance benefits for employees and their dependents—face several disincentives to participating in the financing of long-term care insurance for a primarily retired population. These barriers include tax policies that preclude tax-favored prefunding of any retiree health benefits; enormous unfunded liabilities for retiree acute health care; and increasing pressures for cost containment in the face of skyrocketing health care costs, foreign competition, and employee demands for better compensation packages.

Simultaneously, families are increasingly hard-pressed to provide informal care at home as they juggle to balance the demands of children, jobs for both the husband and wife, and, frequently, geographic distance from elder loved ones. Furthermore, neither elders nor their families can readily afford to purchase needed long-term care services as health care inflation far outpaces the growth in any assets and savings they may have for such a purpose.

Recommendations

Thus it is clear that integrated and complementary programs of public and private financing are needed. Clearly, a purely private financing strategy is not feasible. Neither is a purely public strategy. Regardless of our philosophical predispositions on the role of government, we ought to focus our attention on the design of a financing strategy that includes individuals and their families, employers and insurers, service providers as well as federal and state governments.

Of equal importance, we must recognize that the problem of financing long-term care is not just a financing problem. It is a financing problem, a service delivery problem, a health promotion and research problem, a data collection problem, and a consumer education problem.

After a year of study, of listening, and of learning, the Connecticut Commission on Private and Public Responsibilities for Financing Long Term Care for the Elderly concluded that better methods of public and private financing are needed. The delivery system—particularly community-based services—must be expanded to accommodate growing demands; cost control mechanisms are needed; and long-range preventive measures must be taken to improve the well-being of future generations of elders, to reduce the need for services.

A large-scale, universal entitlement program simply promising an infusion of more money is inappropriate at this time, for several reasons. Private-sector financing alternatives are emerging and represent an affordable alternative for many. The current delivery system is inadequate in both overall capacity and structures to assure appropriate services and placements for a sudden growth in publicly financed patients. Case management as a cost control mechanism is in its infancy, and an inflow of new public funds would precipitate increased utilization of unknown proportion. Existing data on the current use of private and public funds, on lengths of stay in nursing homes, on spend down and transfer of assets, on use of home care, and other issues are inadequate as a basis for projecting future trends. And, of course, how individuals and families would react under a newly designed system of expanded public funding is totally unknown.

Therefore, careful planning and identification of suitable and targeted public and private roles is the necessary course of action to improve the availability of, quality of, access to, and financing for long-term care. This is the time to stop and think, to study and analyze, to experiment and test.

The following recommendations of the Connecticut Commission reflect a need for the development of a more comprehensive approach to the financing issue.

1. *The variety and availability of new methods of private long-term care financing should be increased.* Federal and state governments must, of course, continue to assure access to quality care for those individuals who are unable to provide for themselves.

   The federal and state governments have played and continue to play an important role in providing health care for the elderly. Among other things, government supports nursing home care through the Medicaid program at a cost of approximately $15 billion per year, thereby meeting almost one-half of the nation's nursing home bills for the elderly. Given the projected increase in demand for health care services, however, this level of funding must not only continue but increase, and it must be supplemented by additional federal health care strategies.

   Tax incentives are the most obvious means by which the federal government can encourage private financing of long-term care. Very limited financial incentives currently exist for the private financing of long-term care through savings, insurance, pensions, and family contributions.

   Creating tax incentives and removing tax barriers to new, as well as existing, private methods of financing long-term care will encourage employers, individuals, insurers, and other financial institutions to expand their roles in long-term care.

   In view of the essential role that families play in providing informal care to their elders, the federal government should expand incentives and support for these family efforts. Current tax incentives for family caregiving are very difficult to qualify for because of the restrictive definitions and tests of "dependency." Modifications to the tax code should be made to create incentives for family members to care for their elders.

   In addition to these public strategies, the variety and availability of new methods of private long-term care financing should be increased to meet the demands of diverse market segments and to moderate the increase in pressures on public treasuries at the state and federal level. These methods include home equity conversion, insurance, health maintenance organizations, continuing care retirement communities, and other innovative alternatives. The more private financing options available, the greater will be the opportunity to avoid the negative consequences of the present system—spousal impoverishment, asset transfer, and growing public liability.

154

Fundamentally, individuals must plan ahead for their own long-term care financing needs to the extent they are financially able to do so in their younger years. And families must continue to care for their loved ones to the extent they are able—by both providing informal care and subsidizing the purchase of formal services.

Employers should sponsor and offer long-term care insurance programs to employees and retirees. As improved private insurance products come on the market, employers should make these available either on a shared-cost or employee-pay-all basis.

The federal and state governments should serve as role models to employers by offering long-term care insurance to their employees, retirees, and appropriate dependents.

Government, the states in particular, should nurture, or at least not impede, the development and use of private financing options. For example, in Connecticut the commission found that certain Medicaid eligibility requirements discouraged the use of home equity conversions for financing long-term care and recommended their revision. In addition, the commission recommended the adoption of state regulations enabling the sale of a wide variety of long-term care insurance products. The federal government should look more favorably on applications for Medicare and Medicaid waivers from those states interested in testing new models of long-term care delivery and public/private financing partnerships.

2. *The availability of and financing for home and community based alternatives must be expanded.* These home and community-based services complement and sustain family caregiving efforts and, as an alternative to institutional care, represent savings to the individual, the family, and potentially the public sector.

As financing options are created, available services with appropriate cost controls must also be expanded. We will need to encourage the development of community-based alternatives by expanding Medicaid coverage of services such as adult day care and respite care.

In addition, new techniques for controlling costs and for managing the appropriateness and quality of long-term care services will need to be developed. A national network of quality, professional case managers is an integral element of a cost and utilization control strategy. Such a national network does not now exist. Prescreening and on-going case management for public and private-pay long-term care patients will be needed.

3. *Long-range strategies must be developed to meet and to moderate future demand for services.* Positive long-range strategies should include the extended employment of older adults, disease prevention and health promotion, expanded support of research into the diseases of old age, and expanded support for the training of health care professionals.

Increased financing options and expanded service delivery systems will not be sufficient if we do not simultaneously work to reduce the numbers of elderly who will be in need of long-term care in the future.

4. *Consumer education programs regarding long-term care financing should be expanded.* A more educated population will better understand the need for timely personal financial planning efforts. Furthermore, consumer education, together with an effective program of consumer protection, will enable individuals to make selective, informed choices. As a consequence, traumas such as spousal impoverishment may be reduced and pressure for public support moderated.

5. *Data collection efforts and public dissemination of information regarding long-term care service utilization must be improved.* The lack of data, particularly longitudinal data that describes long-term care service utilization over time, presents design and product-pricing difficulties for government, providers, insurers, and other entities that might provide long-term care risk-sharing products, e.g., health maintenance organizations and continuing care retirement communities.

Information is the key to managing risk, and its availability will therefore expedite the entry into the market of both more products and more product sponsors.

Conclusion

Clearly we are all responsible in some measure for the long-term care needs of our society. Already we all contribute a small amount to long-term care expenses through taxes that support Medicaid and other public programs. In addition, with the rare exception of those few of us who are insured, we all face a risk of exorbitant, devastating long-term care costs, which we will pay for largely out-of-pocket. Last, we all pay the emotional costs of anxiety and exhaustion when we provide care to loved ones, or of guilt and powerlessness when we must watch them become impoverished and stripped of their dignity by long-term care costs.

We have the opportunity to moderate the growth in the amount we pay through the public taxing system by creating better reimbursement and service delivery methods, by improving elderly health status, and even potentially by expanding the total contribution to long-term care expenses derived from the private sector. We also have the opportunity to manage, plan for, and spread the risks of personal financial devastation by promoting the development and use of private financing options.

These opportunities must be aggressively pursued. However, no single sector of society can achieve this alone. The complexities of the long-term care financing issue require a multifaceted response and the participation of all segments of society. Public and private sectors must work together cooperatively to create an integrated, rational system of financing.

XII. Retirement Benefits for University Employees: Evaluating the Tradeoffs[1]

PAPER BY THOMAS O'BRIEN AND RICHARD WOODBURY

Historically, universities have responded to important employee needs by initiating new employee benefit programs or by expanding existing programs. Today, the two principal financial risks facing retirees in higher education are inflation and long-term disability. Universities considering ways to address these issues are discouraged by the high cost of inflation-adjusted pension plans and long-term care insurance plans. This paper discusses how the approach to employee benefit programs might be changed and the plans reorganized to address these important retirement needs.

Employers typically spend between 35 and 40 percent of wages and salaries to provide their employees with retirement benefits, health benefits, paid vacation, holidays and sick leave, Social Security and unemployment contribution, and other benefits. Total employee compensation is allocated between wages and benefits, and among different types of benefits.

Tax laws have a substantial impact on the allocation between wages and benefits. While most wage compensation is fully taxable to the employee, most benefit plans are exempt from taxation. As a result, employees can be better off at a lower cost to employers if compensation is provided through employee benefits.

The allocation among benefits is determined by a combination of employer objectives and employee preferences.

The tradeoffs between insurance benefits and entitlement benefits are particularly relevant and rarely discussed. Insurance benefits are used only by employees with special needs, while entitlement benefits are used by all employees. Retirement benefit programs typically emphasize entitlements rather than insurance. Health plans provide routine care and acute medical care, but not long-term care; dental plans provide check-ups, but not expensive dental procedures; pension plans provide adequate income at retirement, but little inflation protection.

[1] This study was funded in part by a grant from Carnegie Corporation of New York.

159

Alternatively, one could design a system that emphasizes insurance. Retirement health plans in this model would provide complete coverage for expensive medical and long-term care, but would require employees to pay a substantial deductible for smaller medical needs; retirement income would automatically adjust to changes in the cost of living, but the initial income would be smaller. One could also design a retirement program that provides both entitlement benefits and insurance benefits but that requires sacrifices in preretirement wages and salary.

It is not just coincidence that benefit programs emphasize entitlements. Entitlement benefits are extremely popular and their popularity reflects some fundamental aspects of human nature. Insurance plans require the contribution of the many to provide for the supplementary needs of the few. Many people would choose not to make these contributions, since they consider themselves unlikely to experience such supplementary needs. A definite benefit, such as a dental check-up, often seems more attractive than an unlikely benefit, such as dental surgery.

As colleges and universities address the issues of inflation and long-term care, they will need to evaluate the traditional tradeoffs between wages and benefits, and confront directly those between entitlements and insurance. Compensation packages cannot do everything for everyone. What forms of compensation do employees want? How do these differ from what they may need? What common objectives does the institution stand for? This paper considers these issues in the context of a single institution, Harvard University. The issues exist throughout higher education. Indeed, they exist for all employers and are brought into focus by the needs of an aging work force and the prospect for dramatic increases in the number and life expectancy of retirees.

Retirement Benefit Objectives

There are many starting points from which to consider fringe benefits. Three distinct approaches have developed among employers: a market-based approach, a flexible benefit approach, and a corporate philosophy approach.

Using the market-based approach, employers offer fringe benefits as part of a compensation package designed to attract and retain workers. Whether through surveys, collective bargaining, or trial and error, the market signals employers as to what benefits should be included in the compensation package.

The flexible benefit approach emphasizes employee choice. The most simple flexible benefit packages offer employees a choice between two or three benefit variations. More complex cafeteria plans provide employees with a specified number of dollars which can be allocated among alternative benefits or as salary or wage supplements. With a totally flexible approach, the employer is indifferent to whether an employee has health insurance, a retirement pension, or no benefits at all. The employee makes the decision.

Using the corporate philosophy approach, organizations decide on benefits based on what employees "should" receive as part of the corporate package. These decisions may be a simple expression of the chief executive officer's (CEO's) conviction that employees should have a fully paid comprehensive health plan or should have a retirement plan which enables them to retire at age 62. The reality behind such expression is often idiosyncratic to the CEO. The original retirement income plan at Harvard, for example, was a direct result of the interest of President Charles Eliot.

> In the opinion of the President, there is no way in which a given sum of money—like $100,000 or $500,000—can be applied so productively for the University as by making it hasten the time when a thorough system of retiring allowances can be adopted [*Annual Report of the President and Treasurer of Harvard College*, 1898–1899].

Benefit programs based on corporate philosophy can also serve an important social purpose by providing employees with health insurance or retirement savings which they might neglect to provide for themselves. In this way, employers have an important opportunity to communicate their concern for employee welfare, improving worker morale and motivation. Regardless of the origin or motivation behind the corporate philosophy, it is the employer who then decides the quantity and composition of benefits.

Retirement Benefits at Harvard

The evolution of fringe benefits at Harvard has relied on all three approaches. The adequacy of the benefit programs has been evaluated by comparison with the benefits offered by other employers, by their ability to attract and retain desirable employees, by their responsiveness to the needs and desires of individual employees, and by a genuine concern for the lifestyle and financial security of employees.

Although Harvard has responded to the market and to employee desires, corporate philosophy has often led to the implementation of benefit programs more generous than those offered by competing employers. Harvard's initiative in creating a "Retiring Allowance Fund" reflects this concern for the employee's lifestyle and financial security in retirement.

> The chief reasons for the adoption of some good system of retiring annuities in the University are these: First, it would add to the dignity and attractiveness of the service, by securing all participants against the chance of falling into poverty late in life, or of seeing an associate so reduced; secondly, it would provide for participants the means of honorable ease, when the capacity and inclination for work abate; thirdly, it would promote the efficiency of the service by enabling the Corporation, without inflicting hardship, to relieve from active duty officers whose powers are impaired by age ... [*Annual Report of the President and Treasurer of Harvard College*, 1878–1879].

The "Retiring Allowance Fund" enabled Harvard to adopt a program of retirement pensions in 1899.

> The adoption of this system of retiring allowances marks a new epoch for university officials in the United States; for it is the first carefully considered and comprehensive university system to be put in force in the country. It makes the position of a Harvard professor much more desirable than it ever was before; since it secures him after forty-five years of age or thereabouts against every adverse chance except untimely death ... [*Annual Report of the President and Treasurer of Harvard College*, 1898–1899].

Over the past century, the desirability of financial security for retired Harvard employees has led to a gradual increase in retirement benefits. The income replacement rate on pension annuities has risen from roughly 30 percent to more than 70 percent. In 1956, Harvard assumed the entire cost of faculty pensions. The same occurred for staff in 1962. And in 1966, the University began to pay all medical insurance costs for retired employees.

The wholly noncontributory retirement plan was largely motivated by the 1956 Report of the Committee on Compensation (the Bundy Report).

> The single most desirable change in present arrangements, we think, would be a change in our retirement plan for officers of instruction and administration ... We strongly recommend that the University assume the full cost of such retirement contributions ... [Report of the Committee on Compensation, 1956].

The 1968 report of the Committee on Recruitment and Retention of Faculty (the *Dunlop Report*) describes the Harvard retirement plan as "excellent compared to most other university plans."

Harvard has paid a significant price for its expression of corporate philosophy. Fringe benefits which were added because they sounded worthwhile and seemed to have a low cost, such as health coverage for retired employees, have often proven to be quite expensive. Once a benefit is provided, the courts and employee relations make it almost impossible to retract. Health costs, dental costs, and Social Security have combined to add considerable costs to the University's compensation package.

Paying the entire cost of retirement benefits has proved particularly costly. Employers experience significantly lower benefit costs when a portion of these costs is paid by employees. Cost sharing has important effects on both per employee costs and on the overall level of employee participation in benefit programs. In health insurance, for example, it pays couples to select only one insurance plan when both are employed if there is a charge to the employee for insurance. Deductibles and copayments induce employees to be more conservative in their use of medical services. Consequently, employers with some form of cost sharing have significantly lower participation and lower costs per employee than employers without cost sharing. Pension plans which require matching contributions from employees can also have significantly less than full employee participation.

Harvard is now considering the issue of whether to provide more protection from inflation and long-term disability. As with any employee benefits, tradeoffs are essential. The expenditure required for an inflation adjusted pension plan or a long-term care insurance plan could be used for wages and salaries, for other employee benefits, or for any category of university expenditure.

Health and Long-Term Care Benefits

Health insurance is intended to protect employees from the financial risk of accident and serious illness. Most health insurance programs also provide assistance with more routine medical expenses. Herzlinger and Schwartz identify this dual function:

Health care insurance is unusual among insurance programs. Unlike other forms of insurance—life, disability, workmen's compensation—it does not protect solely against severe financial dislocations in people's lives. Some of the expenses health insurance covers are for small items;

163

for example, 25 percent of health insurance benefits in 1980 were paid for annual expenses of less than $1,000, and only 40 percent were for major annual expenses exceeding $5,000. It's like using homeowner's insurance for routine home maintenance rather than for major liabilities. And, of course, the costs of providing the present low deductible and low coinsurance form of health insurance are high (Herzlinger and Schwartz, 1985).

The combination of Medicare and Medigap insurance offered to almost all retired Harvard employees provides generous medical care benefits. At the same time, however, retired employees with long-term disabilities receive no assistance with nursing home or home health care expenses.

Medicare alone covers about 49 percent of the medical care expenses for the elderly population. With "catastrophic care" legislation, out-of-pocket expenditures for Medicare-covered services will be limited. The new limit, along with the deductible and copayment features of the Medicare program, make it an insurance benefit—people pay for their initial medical care, but are fully covered for more serious medical needs.

Medex III, which is paid for by Harvard for its retirees, covers the deductibles and copayments of the Medicare program. Particularly with a cap on out-of-pocket expenditures for Medicare covered services, Medex is much more of an entitlement benefit. Medex provides first dollar medical coverage which will be used by everyone, not just those most in need.

Together, Medicare and Medex provide up to 365 days of hospital charges and inpatient physician charges (120 days in a mental hospital), some private duty nursing services for inpatients, up to 100 days of skilled nursing home care, most emergency outpatient care, and most prescription drug expenses. Some of these provisions require the use of Medicare or Blue Cross-Blue Shield approved providers to receive the full benefit. Harvard retirees also have the use of the University Health Services for consultations, routine office visits, and physical examinations. A few retired employees choose to enroll in HMO-sponsored senior plans, with similar benefits.

While Harvard's medical care coverage is extensive, its long-term care coverage is not. The single greatest risk to the financial security of a retired Harvard employee is long-term disability. Neither Medicare nor Medigap policies cover long-term care expenses, no major employer currently provides long-term care benefits, and private long-term care insurance is effectively unavailable.

A Commission on College Retirement and a Commission on Long-

Term Care have begun to explore the long-term care needs of retired university employees. According to their reports, the risks of long-term disability are substantial.

In 1982, an estimated 4.3 million older people, about 17 percent of the population over age 65, experienced disabilities that made it difficult to carry out activities of daily living such as eating, washing, or dressing without the assistance of another individual . . .

The proportion of the elderly needing personal care assistance increases rapidly with age. Less than 3 percent of those between 65 and 69 years of age need assistance. By age 75 to 79, however, that figure rises to about 10 percent. Finally, about one-third of the elderly above age 85 need personal assistance. Many more elderly need mobility and household assistance [Commission on Long-Term Care, May 1987].

While some long-term care needs are provided informally by family and friends, others are provided professionally, through nursing homes or home health care organizations. These long-term care services can impose a serious financial burden on the unfortunate people with very long-term disabilities. Since Medicare covers almost no nursing home costs, most people pay nursing home expenses personally until they deplete their wealth and become eligible for means-tested Medicaid assistance. The Commission on Long-Term Care reports these cost statistics for nursing home care alone:

- There is about a 40 percent chance that a 65-year-old will enter a nursing home before death . . . .

- The average expected lifetime costs for a 65-year-old nursing home entrant are about $36,000 . . . . The distribution of costs for nursing home users is highly skewed . . . .

- About 33 percent of nursing home entrants stay longer than one year in a nursing home. For these nursing home entrants, the costs of care can range from between $50,000 to $200,000 (Commission on Long-Term Care, May 1987).

Harvard is evaluating the possibility of offering a long-term care insurance plan in partnership with the Prudential Insurance Company. One proposal would provide long-term care benefits to all retired employees and their spouses, plus all active employees eligible for early retirement. The plan would use a cost reimbursement approach, similar to conventional health insurance plans, providing 80 percent of nursing home expenses up to $70 per day or 80 percent of home health care expenses up to $35 per day. To receive the benefits,

165

employees must satisfy a 90-day waiting period, during which they pay the full cost of care, and they must need assistance from others in two or more of the standard activities of daily living.

This proposal is just one of many possible designs for a long-term care insurance plan. Since long-term care insurance is a young industry, there are many issues which need to be resolved. How much benefit is appropriate? Should insurance cover the cost of room and board in a nursing home? Should there be a difference in benefits if a spouse maintains a separate residence? Should premiums be charged for spousal coverage? How much should beneficiaries be required to pay to prevent the overuse of insured long-term care services? Should the amount of benefit depend on the length of employment? Should long-term care benefits be portable? Should long-term care insurance be integrated with postretirement health insurance?

The integration of acute and long-term care could lower the cost of both benefits, but integration can only be assured by limiting retirees' choice of doctors and treatment. There is considerable discussion about a managed care approach to all medical and custodial care needs. The managed care provider would receive a fixed fee per patient, encouraging providers to contain health care costs. Each individual would be assigned to a managed care counselor, who would diagnose the specific needs of the patient and determine the appropriate mix of health and custodial care services. When appropriate, home health care could replace expensive nursing home care. Nursing home care could replace even more expensive hospital care. The total cost of both medical and long-term care could be substantially reduced.

Regardless of the design, long-term care is an insurance-type benefit. Only retired employees with very long-term disabilities would receive assistance, while the cost of the benefits would be borne by all employees. Moreover, long-term care insurance is very expensive—perhaps as expensive as all other health care benefits combined.

Actuarial estimates vary substantially. The cost of providing the insurance and funding the past service liabilities for retirees, spouses, current employees, and spouses is estimated to be as much as 5 percent of payroll over 30 years. The cost of providing such a benefit would be cut in half if one took a "social insurance" approach, i.e., decided to provide current funding only and continued to postpone funding the past service liability. Uncertainty about future costs makes these estimates very imprecise. It will require significant experience with a plan to arrive at actuarial estimates that do not present an individual employer with the possibility of large cost increases.

The tradeoffs involved in long-term care insurance plan are complex. Employees would sacrifice current salary and benefits in return for retirement benefits. Employees who leave the university before retirement would subsidize those who stay to receive long-term care insurance. Younger employees would subsidize older employees and those already retired. High-income employees would subsidize low-income employees. Most importantly, the many healthy employees and retirees would subsidize the few disabled retirees.

Not all retired employees need long-term care insurance. Those with large wealth or retirement income can pay for extended nursing home care or home health care without impoverishment. Those with little wealth or retirement income receive Medicaid assistance for long-term care. It is the large group of people between the rich and poor who benefit most from long-term care insurance, and this group tends not to realize its vulnerability until a long-term disability occurs.

There is also tremendous uncertainty surrounding the long-term care issue. As federal and state governments begin to explore long-term care needs, it is unclear what benefits will be provided publicly and what tax and regulatory rules will affect private long-term care programs. It is unclear how much long-term care services will cost when active employees reach the age when they need such services. It is unclear what new technologies will develop to deal with long-term disabilities. It is unclear to what extent long-term care insurance will increase the use of long-term care services.

Given the high cost, the politically unpopular tradeoffs, and the uncertainties surrounding long-term care, why would any employer consider long-term care insurance? The answer falls in the category of corporate philosophy. Long-term care costs are a major threat to income security in retirement. The unfunded liability for Harvard's current retirees and spouses is estimated to be $40 million. These costs will occur with or without insurance. It is inefficient for individuals to save for the small possibility that they will be subject to catastrophic long-term care expenses. Insurance in the private market is expensive and largely unexplored. If the employer truly cares about income security in retirement, then some sort of employer-sponsored long-term care insurance is essential.

There is also a flexible benefit approach to long-term care which is being considered at the University of California (UC)—a completely voluntary and employee-paid plan. While this would be a significant improvement over no long-term care plan, there is reason to expect that very few people would elect to participate. As a result, there would still be many retirees without protection from the financial risk of long-term disability.

The real issue is evaluating the tradeoffs. Health insurance plans with first-dollar coverage are more expensive and more popular than those without first-dollar coverage. The savings from an elimination of first-dollar benefits could be used to provide more insurance from financial risks. Do universities have an institutional responsibility to protect retired employees from the financial risk of long-term disability? What do employees want and what are the institutional goals?

Retirement Income

Many similar issues and objectives, such as the distinction between insurance and entitlement benefits, are also relevant to the design of a retirement income plan. The value of the entitlement benefit is best determined by comparing retirement income with preretirement income. According to the booklet that describes the pension plan, "At Harvard, the university's objective is to provide a person who has at least 25 years of service at normal retirement with an after-tax income, from both the Harvard pension and Social Security combined, of 70 percent to 80 percent of net salary (after taxes) during the final year before retirement" (pension description booklet). This replacement rate is usually sufficient for retired employees to maintain their standard of living during the early years of retirement.

> Retirees require considerably less than 100 percent of their preretirement income to maintain their standard of living. Whereas preretirement earnings are subject to the federal income tax, the Social Security payroll tax, and state and municipal income taxes, a large portion of retirement income is not taxed. . .
> Second, work-related expenses, such as transportation, clothing, and meals purchased away from home, are reduced during retirement. Pension contributions and other saving can also cease in retirement [Commission on College Retirement, May 1986].

The initial replacement ratio, however, may not be sufficient to protect retired employees from the financial risks of inflation. Unlike Social Security payments, most private retirement annuities are not adjusted for changes in the cost of living. Harvard staff automatically receive a fixed income retirement annuity. Faculty select an annuity from the alternatives offered by TIAA/CREF (Teachers Insurance and Annuity Association and College Retirement Equities Fund), and most faculty also choose a fixed income annuity. Harvard has periodically provided pension increases to retirees, but these increases are not part of the retirement plan and do not fully offset the effects of inflation.

> Maintaining living standards over the entire period of retirement requires not only establishing an adequate initial benefit but also protecting the benefit from the effects of inflation. In an inflationary environment, the purchasing power of benefits fixed in nominal terms will deteriorate and retirees' standards of living will decline. When high rates of inflation are combined with earlier retirement and increased longevity, the value of unindexed pension benefits falls drastically. Even a relatively mild rate of inflation, such as 4 percent, will cut the purchasing power nearly in half over a 15-year period. [Commission on College Retirement, May 1986].

A standard measure of inflation, such as the Consumer Price Index (CPI), may not be the best index of inflation for the products purchased by retired university employees. At Harvard, for example, most retired employees own their home and receive free medical care, so inflation in the price of housing and medical care would not affect their cost of living. Over the past decade, the average annual inflation rate for housing and medical care exceeded the average overall inflation rate by 1.7 and 2.1 percent, respectively. As a result, the CPI probably overestimates the appropriate inflation index.

While the current staff and faculty pension plans at Harvard have the same retirement income objectives, they have very different approaches. The staff have a defined benefit plan: the size of the pension depends on the final salary of the employee and the number of years of Harvard employment. The faculty have a defined contribution plan in which Harvard contributes a certain percentage of salary to a tax-exempt investment account (TIAA or CREF): the size of the pension depends on how much savings has accumulated in that account.

Universities need to evaluate the tradeoffs inherent in these two approaches. If the only objective is to provide an income replacement rate of 70 to 80 percent, then a defined benefit plan is more efficient than a defined contribution plan. First, a defined contribution plan provides a higher than intended income replacement rate for faculty who choose a later retirement. For each additional year of employment, employers must continue to contribute to the retirement account, the existing assets in the account continue to accumulate, and the expected number of years of retirement decreases. As a result, some faculty receive retirement income which actually exceeds their preretirement salary.

169

Second, faculty automatically receive any "overfunding" in the defined contribution plan. If the retirement assets earn a particularly high rate of return, then retirees automatically receive a higher pension annuity. "Overfunding" in the defined benefit plan could be used to provide other benefits, rather than to supplement an already adequate retirement income.

Third, pension savings tend to be invested in assets with a higher rate of return in a defined benefit plan than in a defined contribution plan. Under the defined contribution plan at Harvard, more retirement savings have been invested in the low risk fixed income TIAA account than in the higher risk variable income CREF account, despite the fact that CREF historically offers a higher average rate of return. Under the defined benefit plan, pension investments are managed by Harvard, and Harvard has earned a higher rate of return than typical TIAA and CREF accounts. As a result, the prefunded cost of any retirement annuity is lower in the defined benefit plan than in the defined contribution plan.

In addition to the cost inefficiencies of the defined contribution plan, its retirement age sensitivity creates a large financial incentive not to retire. Furthermore, beginning in 1993, universities can no longer require faculty retirement at age 70. This could lead to some faculty members staying far beyond their most productive years, for purely financial reasons. Biggs makes the following observation about a typical defined contribution plan with contributions continuing until actual retirement.

- The rise in retirement incomes from age 65 to 70 is remarkable—a 130-percent increase in this illustration. Surely many participants will find this a powerful financial incentive to stay in the work force.

- The more-than-doubling effect continues in each 5-year period—the participant could look forward to an income more than 10 times as great at age 80 than at age 65.

- Although the retirement-income-to salary ratio is not too bad at age 70, no reasonable rationale for life-cycle income support can argue for the design of a pension that produces such retirement income/salary patterns at age 75—let alone the extraordinary case of age 80. Should one project further to ages 85 and 90? [Biggs, 1983].

Despite its drawbacks, the defined contribution plan is very popular among university faculty. The defined contribution plan allows employees to see and control their retirement savings more directly; it allows some faculty to receive a higher than expected pension annuity; and it allows easy portability of retirement savings. Faculty committees have consistently expressed their support for a defined contribution approach.

It is clear that no single investment plan for pension contributions is ideal for all faculty members. They differ in their expectations of price changes in the future, in the proportion which accumulated pension contributions constitute of total assets, in the distribution of other assets, and in their willingness to assume risks in equities. The opportunity to choose among alternative plans, provided their comparative features and consequences are well understood, is an advantage to the faculty as a whole [1968 Report of the Committee on Recruitment and Retention of Faculty].

The Committee believes that it is better to continue the pension system on the basis which it now has, namely, that the actual pension in each case depends upon the amount of payment made over the years for each individual faculty member, these payments being a percentage of salary. This gives full recognition to the idea that the pension payments are related to the worth of services rendered at Harvard [1949 Report of Faculty Committee on Academic Pensions].

While slightly more difficult administratively, portability can be incorporated into a defined benefit plan. The current staff plan, for example, offers some portability:

The new portable benefit formula provides a single lump sum amount which is generally payable in cash when you leave the University before age 55. The lump sum benefit is designed to provide a "portable" sum that you can invest on your own or in another employer's plan until you do retire.

The Commission on College Retirement suggests that the portable benefits in defined benefit plans be even more generous:

There are a number of ways to eliminate the discrimination of defined benefit plans against mobile employees . . . [E]ither the pension received in retirement should be based on a salary projected to the time of retirement (rather than the salary at the time of job severance) or an amount of cash necessary to fund such a benefit should be rolled over into the new employer's retirement plan. Such cash rollovers would amount to a sum similar to what would have accumulated in an equivalent defined contribution plan [Commission on College Retirement, May 1986].

An interesting alternative would be a defined benefit plan with a defined contribution underlay. The defined benefit plan would apply to employees who retire from an institution. The defined contribution underlay would be a fully portable individual pension account available to any employee who leaves. The plan would be designed so that the payments under the defined benefit plan would always be larger than the annuity payments possible from the defined contribution account. This hybrid plan could have all the advantages of a defined benefit plan, with the high portability of a defined contribution plan.

Again, the real issue is evaluating the tradeoffs. A defined contribution plan is more expensive and more popular than a defined benefit plan. The savings from a defined benefit plan could be used to provide more insurance from financial risks. Do universities have an institutional responsibility to protect retired employees from the financial risk of inflation? What do employees want and what are the institutional goals?

Retirement Benefit Integration

This discussion has consistently encouraged the evaluation of tradeoffs. Specifically, what tradeoffs might be available to protect retired employees from the financial risks of inflation and long-term disability? Some of the cost might be paid for with salary reductions. Some savings might be found by trading off first-dollar health coverage. Some savings might be found by integrating acute and long-term care. Some savings might be found by using a defined benefit approach to faculty pensions.

If an employer chooses to trade off entitlement benefits and to promote insurance and financial security, an integrated approach to retirement benefits could result in additional savings. A single program of retirement security would include inflation protection and a health insurance plan covering both acute and long-term care. The cost savings would result from the sharing of funds. Any surpluses in one aspect of the retirement program could automatically compensate for deficits in another aspect of the program.

The economies of this approach are best evaluated by comparison with current retirement plans. Many defined contribution retirement accounts are large enough to support a retirement annuity larger than preretirement salary. Many defined benefit plans are also overfunded. What should these surplus funds be used for? Surpluses in defined contribution accounts are automatically converted to higher faculty pensions.

While rarely evaluated in this context, these surpluses could also be used to provide more insurance from financial risks. Excess reserves in the staff and faculty pension plans could be used to fund part of the cost of long-term care insurance premiums. Old life insurance policies could be rolled over into long-term care insurance policies as the need for life insurance decreases.

Summary

Long-term care needs and the risks of inflation are unlikely to be met simply by increased benefit contributions. The cost would be very high. Confronted with the high cost of inflation-adjusted pensions and long-term care insurance, employers should step back and evaluate their benefit plans. Have they chosen the right mix of salary, entitlement benefits, and insurance benefits? How might benefit programs be changed to improve the mix? What forms of compensation do employees want and what risks do employers wish to assume? The debate may be as important as its results.

References

Biggs, John H. "Designing Pension Plans to Incorporate Recent Legislation." *Educational Record* (Summer 1983): 32–36.

Commission on College Retirement. *A Pension Program for College and University Personnel.* New York, NY: Commission on College Retirement, 1986.

Commission on College Retirement. *A Plan to Create Comprehensive Group Long-Term Care Insurance For College and University Personnel.* Discussion draft. New York, NY: Commission on College Retirement, 1986.

Commission on Long-Term Care. *Long-Term Care: Three Approaches to University-Based Insurance.* New York, NY: Commission on Long Term Care, 1987.

Commission on Long-Term Care. *Understanding How to Evaluate the Structure and Administration of University or College-Based Long-Term Care Insurance.* New York, NY: Commission on Long Term Care, 1987. Draft.

Harris, Seymour E. *The Economics of Harvard.* New York, NY: McGraw-Hill Book Company, 1970.

Harvard College. *Annual Report of the President and Treasurer of Harvard College.* (1878–1879, 1898–1899). Cambridge, MA: Harvard College, 1879–1899.

Harvard University. *Report of Faculty Committee on Academic Pensions.* Cambridge, MA: Harvard University, 1949.

Harvard University. *Report of the Committee on Compensation.* Cambridge, MA: Harvard University, 1956.

Harvard University. *Report of the Committee on the Recruitment and Retention of Faculty.* Cambridge, MA: Harvard University, 1968.

Herzlinger, R. E., and J. Schwartz. "How Companies Tackle Health Care Costs." *Harvard Business Review* 4 (July-August 1985).

XIII. Long-Term Care: Feasibility of Employer Involvement

PAPER BY JOHN J. MCCORMACK

Pressures on Employers

Employers are under extraordinary pressure as benefit providers. Starting in 1974 with ERISA (Employee Retirement Income Security Act) through to the Tax Reform Act of 1986, they have been hit with an onslaught of legislation. Regulations from the federal and state level have forced employers to extend and make changes to benefits for employees. On top of that, the skyrocketing medical CPI has made it necessary for employers to exercise cost-containment measures on most health insurance plans. And, as the life expectancy in the United States continues to increase, further pressure will be imposed on existing medical insurance plans. The aging of the population has also focused attention on the need to provide for the cost of long-term care—a need which is currently unmet in any planned or organized way.

Today, about 6.6 million, or one in four, Americans over the age of 65 need long-term care. And as the number of older people, particularly those over age 85, continues to increase, it is predicted that by 2040 the number of persons needing care will climb to 19 million. The bulk of the cost for long-term care is paid for out-of-pocket. When income and savings are depleted, most people depend on Medicaid. As a possible solution to this pressing problem, employer-sponsored plans seem to hold great promise.

Given the current environment facing employers as benefit providers, how likely is it that they are in a position to provide a new and relatively expensive benefit? Is it feasible for employers to help with the solution to this pressing social and economic need? With the government mandates on employers in recent years, I think it is likely that employers are going to *have* to provide solutions. It can no longer be a question of whether, but *how* and *when* employer-sponsored long-term care plans will be widely available.

Both federal and state governments are looking for ways to reduce their outlays for medical care expenditures and are, therefore, looking to private initiatives for providing long-term care insurance. Employer-sponsored plans hold the promise of being able to offer long-term care products at a lower cost and therefore of having the greatest impact on Medicaid costs with a consequent reduction in government spending. Furthermore, if the private sector does not initiate solutions, it may, at some time in the future, be required by state or federal requirements to provide long-term care benefits. If it comes down to government mandates, employers could lose control and flexibility in structuring their programs and providing a benefit could ultimately be more costly without that control.

Advantages of Employer-Sponsored Programs

There are several advantages to providing long-term care through employer-sponsored programs. Employer-sponsored group plans are the predominant way current health insurance products are provided in this country. The employer role in private insurance can be traced back to the post-World War II era when, through collective bargaining, employees began to look beyond financial compensation. They sought protection from the costs of catastrophic events such as premature death, disability, and unexpected illness. Employer needs resulting from collective bargaining agreements, the need to compete for employees, and preferential tax treatment of employer benefits are major reasons for the rapid growth and success of the private insurance system in this country over the last 30 or more years.

The next logical step in the evolution of employer-sponsored group plans is protection against the cost of long-term care. The advantages of employer involvement are clear. Through group products, the cost of providing insurance is lower because, with the inclusion of a younger population in premium payments, the actuarial risk is spread over a longer period. Also, as a means of paying for benefits, payroll deduction is usually more acceptable than out-of-pocket payments. When employers sponsor long-term care coverage, it can be offered as an add-on to an existing medical plan or integrated with other forms of group insurance or pension plans. The add-on approach is particularly workable as part of increasingly popular cafeteria plans. Integration of long-term care benefits with other medical programs offers the advantage of greater efficiency in monitoring and administering benefits through a continuum of care, if that is an employer goal.

Employers are also in a unique position to increase awareness and educate large numbers of people about the need for long-term care. Employer communication is just about the best way to reach younger employees who may be most unaware of the risk involved in having no or insufficient coverage for long-term care. Employers can also offer employees an added degree of consumer protection, because the benefits personnel who deal with the insurance companies are experienced in selecting sound and reliable insurance products.

This situation has an advantage over an individual insurance approach to long-term care coverage, which might be aimed at people who are elderly, frail and, in many cases, uninformed purchasers of insurance products.

While employer-sponsored plans seem to hold the greatest degree of promise at this time, they are not being encouraged to the exclusion of other initiatives such as medical IRAs (Individual Retirement Accounts), home equity conversion, and continuing care communities. Endeavors such as these are important because they increase our options. However, these concepts are new and, in many cases, unexplored territory. Through the success of employer-sponsored group insurance over the last few decades, we know that it works. The public trusts and depends on benefits provided by employers. Right now the responsibility for the fastest and most efficient expansion of long-term care insurance rests with employers.

Lack of Availability of Employer Plans

Why then, it seems logical to ask, are employer plans not more widely available? Many obstacles must be removed before long-term care becomes a widespread employer-sponsored benefit. Obvious among them is the pressure employers are already facing in terms of medical care cost and government mandates regulating benefit plans. Another problem is the scarcity of long-term care products available from insurance companies.

Up until recently, insurance companies were, for the most part, trying to overcome the following barriers:

- *Lack of consumer awareness.* Employees are often confused about the extent of coverage provided by their current retiree health plans or by Medicare. Education is essential because the people do not perceive their risk. They think they are protected by Medicare and other plans, and they are not. It is obviously difficult to sell a product or service to individuals who are either unaware that they need the service or convinced that their need will be met in some other way.

- *Lack of relevant data.* There are insufficient data available at this time for insurance companies to determine either the demand for long-term care services or their cost. Without sufficient information to predict

177

utilization or cost patterns, it is difficult for an insurance company (or an employer) either to design benefits or to set premiums.

- *Legislative and regulatory uncertainty.* Existing law, which was designed for traditional health care products, does not provide sufficient flexibility to deal with long-term care products.

Barriers to Providing Long-Term Care through Employer Plans

Other barriers to providing long-term care through employer-sponsored programs include the following:

- Because of the experimental nature of long-term care policies, there may be a need to adjust the benefits as experience evolves. Recent court decisions have placed in question an employer's ability to reduce benefits for retirees. Conflicting court decisions may even cause employers to reconsider whether they will continue to provide the level of medical coverage they currently offer, let alone provide far less predictable long-term care benefits.

- Recent studies by the Department of Labor indicate that the level of prefunding for existing retiree benefits is inadequate—that significant liabilities are currently unfunded. These liabilities will grow as the ratio of retirees to active workers grows. The tax provisions of the Deficit Reduction Act of 1984 (DEFRA), however, discourage employers from prefunding retiree health benefits by limiting the amount an employer may deduct as reserves and taxing the earnings on those reserves.

- Changes currently being considered by the Financial Accounting Standards Board (FASB) will require that the liability for most retirement benefits be reflected on employers' balance sheets. Including these large unfunded liabilities will significantly weaken those balance sheets. Under these circumstances, employers may be hesitant to assume additional liabilities such as those related to providing long-term care.

- Primary responsibility for the medical costs of older workers has been shifted from Medicare to the employer. This responsibility has created additional costs to employers as well as uncertainty as to what additional cost shifts employers may have to assume in the future.

Overcoming the Hurdles

While these barriers are significant, they do not overshadow the promise of employer involvement. Progress has already been made toward overcoming these hurdles. Several national data bases on long-term care are becoming available to the private sector, which should help product design. The Department of Health and Human Services (HHS) sponsored a technical conference in May 1987 to communicate the contents of these data bases and explain ways that they can best be used. The HHS has released a report which promotes employer sponsorship and offers guidelines for employers. The National Association of Insurance Commissioners (NAIC) has facilitated state legislation and regulation appropriate to these unique insurance products by adopting model legislation that has already been enacted in several states and is being actively considered in a number of others. Such models may establish the framework for state legislation and regulation that will enhance the growth of long-term care products.

The Health Insurance Association of America (HIAA) has undertaken a number of initiatives to address the consumer awareness problem. These include: the establishment of a toll-free telephone service for the elderly to inquire about the availability of insurance coverage; development of a comprehensive long-term care package for its member companies; production of a "Consumer's Guide to Long-Term Care," which has been endorsed by both the AARP and the Department of Health and Human Services; and sponsorship of educational seminars on this topic. The HIAA also recently established an ad hoc committee to study consumer protection issues. And formal gatherings for information sharing are becoming more frequent.

To encourage availability of employer-sponsored long-term care insurance, there is a need for tax incentives at the federal level, which clarify the tax status of this insurance and remove barriers to several logical and effective product designs. Specifically, the incentives for employers to prefund retiree health benefits that were removed by DEFRA should be restored. This would mean amending tax laws specifically to allow full employer deductions for reserves, including medical cost inflation, and also to allow the tax-free buildup of interest on long-term care reserves.

Right now, lack of consumer awareness may be one of the most important hurdles we will have to overcome. For long-term care to be widely implemented by employers, there will need to be a broad endorsement by employers and a willingness to trade off other employer-provided benefits or compensation. And with resources limited, it is employee awareness of the potential costs of long-term care and willingness to participate in its funding that are the key to the ultimate success of employer-sponsored long-term care products.

Beginning Efforts by Employers

Recently, some employers have begun to offer coverage. From the experience of these pioneering companies other employers will gain the information they need to structure group long-term care plans effectively. Each venture into the marketplace provides the industry with additional information on feasibility and viability of private long-term care insurance. This is not unlike the early experience of medical and disability insurance.

Although in its infancy, long-term care insurance is beginning to grow. According to an April 1987 study by HHS, 20 insurance companies are offering plans, insuring 423,000 people. Among these pioneering efforts is an optional long-term care benefit for the retired employees of the state of Alaska, underwritten by Aetna. The coverage will supplement the existing Aetna health insurance program for active and retired Alaska employees. The Travelers Insurance Companies have begun to offer its employees long-term care benefits, fully financed by employees, that include nursing home, custodial, and adult day care. Prudential has a group arrangement with AARP under which a nursing home and home health care benefit has been marketed by mail to members of the association. A privately insured long-term care plan for federal employees is also in the planning stages.

Among these fledgling plans is TIAA's extended care benefit. Thirty-one years ago, TIAA recognized the need to provide for catastrophic health costs with the introduction of its major medical plan. At that time, the need for such coverage was largely unmet. TIAA was one of the first in the major medical arena. And now, years later, in keeping with our philosophy of providing complete and reliable benefit coverage for members of the educational community, we have developed an extended care benefit.

The TIAA coverage is an employer-sponsored nursing home and home health care benefit offered as an add-on to our group major medical plan. The benefit pays 80 percent of the cost of confinement in a skilled or intermediate nursing home or home health care, up to a maximum of $100,000. The plan gives employers in the educational community the flexibility to determine whether to offer the long-term care benefit to all employees or only to older employees or retirees and their dependents. The extended care benefit, which is offered only as part of the major medical plan, offers employers the flexibility to pay for the benefit or make it an employee-pay-all product, and to determine the period of coverage and the daily coverage amount that best suits their needs.

In developing the benefit, we attempted to maintain a balance between filling the real long-term care financing needs of individuals and operating in new uncharted territory. We decided that we would have a copayment because we believe it is important that individuals be aware of their costs so that they will be encouraged to choose the most appropriate and cost-effective care.

Because of the lack of data and the uncertainty of the risk involved, we believe it is prudent initially to include an overall limit on extended care coverage. This can be increased or eliminated over time as we gain more experience. The maximum is designed to provide approximately 5 years of coverage in an average nursing home. (If the plan provides up to $70 in covered charges per day at 80 percent for 5 years, the plan would reach the $100,000 maximum towards the end of the fifth year.) Of course, this could be substantially longer for people who use less expensive covered nursing homes or who can be cared for at home and do not require full-time assistance by home health aides. We selected a maximum that would cover over 90 percent of the nursing stays in the United States. Therefore, such a maximum does, for the vast majority of people, eliminate the prospect of depleting their assets and relying on Medicaid and their families.

TIAA is active in industry associations and the HIAA Task Force on Long-Term Care in particular. Through this involvement we are able to share information we have gained over the last three years as we developed our benefit. We plan to continue to share information with others interested in offering employer-sponsored group plans, as we expand and improve our extended care benefit, in an effort to further encourage employer sponsorship. As other employers and insurers do the same, and as they carry on the commitment to providing employees with protection from the costs of catastrophic life events, employer sponsorship holds fertile ground for addressing one of the most important health care issues we face today.

XIV. The Optimal Role for the Federal Government in Financing Catastrophic and Long-Term Care

PAPER BY ROBERT M. BALL

Introduction

The optimal federal role in financing catastrophic medical care costs and long-term care costs should be to cover these risks under Medicare.* If later on a basic health plan covering acute care for all individuals is adopted, catastrophic and long-term care should be included as well.

In the short term, the federal government might require that catastrophic protection (acute, but not long-term care) be a part of any employer-provided group health insurance plan covering current workers.

It would, however, not be equitable for the federal government to establish a universal health insurance plan covering the risk of large acute care expenses only. While such coverage would be valuable for those who can meet most expenses out of pocket or who already have protection against basic health care costs, it would do little or nothing for the great majority of the approximately 50 million persons who currently either have no health insurance or very inadequate insurance. A health insurance plan covering only the risk of large expenditures would mean taking money from everyone largely for the benefit of those who are already relatively well-off. Those with low incomes, while required to contribute, would be unable to pay large deductibles, which are an inherent part of catastrophic plans.

On the other hand, if one is already covered for basic care costs, catastrophic coverage is an important add-on. Thus, for the Medicare population, or for those of working age with basic insurance, the addition of catastrophic acute care protection and long-term care insurance is desirable. Adding such protection to Medicare makes sense, not just for older people and the disabled but also for their sons and daughters who, in the absence of such a program, have been

---

*Editor's note: The Medicare Catastrophic Coverage Act of 1988 covers an unlimited number of hospital days for covered services but does not provide for long-term care in a nursing home (see Appendix C).

183

struggling more or less alone with the difficult problem of how to provide care for disabled parents.

Catastrophic Insurance

A Fixed Dollar Threshold—At least as long ago as the early 1960s, and probably much earlier, some people argued that instead of a basic plan like Medicare, the government should propose a plan that reimbursed cost only above some level of expenditures, such as $2,000 or $3,000 a year. This view was widely held by staff in the organization that preceded the Office of Management and Budget, the Bureau of the Budget. The reasoning was that people could afford regular and routine costs and that the concern of insurance, particularly a government plan, should be for the very high expenditures that occur for relatively few. Since then, plans have been introduced in Congress from time to time to provide such catastrophic protection for the whole population.

The trouble with this approach is that what seems like a manageable expense to middle and higher income people can be a disaster for those with lower incomes. Such plans would serve mainly the interests of the better-off. This is not the sort of goal the federal government should be pursuing.

Threshold Defined as a Percentage of Income—Since a fixed dollar threshold has the fatal flaw of helping most those who are already the best off, why not a plan which defines catastrophe in terms of a percentage of family income? Such a definition is clearly better for analytical purposes, as it measures the ability to handle a given level of expenditures in a way that a fixed dollar threshold does not. Although better analytically, in my view, it is not a good way to design specifications for an operating program.

It has seemed to most Americans quite acceptable in a public insurance program to differentiate *contributions* by income. This is true of payroll taxes generally and very conspicuously in the hospital insurance part of Medicare. In this program, the $40,000 worker pays four times as much as the $10,000 worker for exactly the same benefits.[1]

On the other hand, the welfare principle of differentiating *benefits* by current income at the time of receipt fundamentally changes the

---

[1] For 1987, the employee contribution for Hospital Insurance coverage under Medicare was 1.45 percent of earnings up to a maximum of $43,800. As a result, a worker with taxable earnings of $40,000 would contribute $450 annually, while the worker with earnings of $10,000 would pay only $135.

way people react to a program. Tying benefits to an individual demonstration of an inadequate current income, with its overt penalty on savers, destroys the concept of an earned right based on past contributions and previous wages. I doubt if people would accept a contributory system in which the high contributor gets a lower benefit than the low contributor.

There are other problems. The administration of income tests is costly and fraught with difficulty. Moreover, there is an inherent dilemma about where to set the minimum deductible. If the lowest deductible is set at a relatively high income level, the program becomes a health plan covering most people. Such a plan would be almost as expensive as universal health insurance, but would have the disadvantages of an income test. It is much more likely that a catastrophic plan with income-related deductibles would provide low deductibles only for those with very low incomes and high deductibles for the average person. This is the usual model, and it leaves much of the problem unsolved.

The conclusion is that catastrophic acute care coverage is best implemented with a fixed dollar deductible, but only as an add-on to basic insurance protection. It is appropriate then to add such protection to group insurance for current workers and to Medicare.

Improving Catastrophic Protection under Medicare—Following the passage of the Medicare Catastrophic Coverage Act of 1988, Medicare beneficiaries will still have to contend with costs that for many will be disastrous. They will still have to pay a high hospital deductible, a high drug benefit deductible, the Part B deductible, higher Part B premiums, payments to physicians who charge more than Medicare will approve as a basis for reimbursement, and the 20 percent co-payment in Part B. They will have to make up for the failure to cover dental care and most preventive services, along with hearing aids and eye glasses. Even so, substantial progress will have been made if the current proposals become law. It is quite proper that the emphasis should now shift to what has all along been the truly catastrophic cost for Medicare beneficiaries and their families: long-term care.

Long-Term Care Insurance

The Unique Character of Long-Term Care—Like catastrophic acute care, long-term care can result in huge costs, but there the resemblance ends. Long-term care is most commonly associated with personal care services rendered over a long period of time to people who need help with the activities of daily living, such as eating, dressing, bathing, going to the toilet, and moving from one place to another, or who need constant supervison because of mental impairment. On the other hand, catastrophic acute care costs usually arise from a medical episode or series of episodes which require the use of hospitals, physicians and, frequently, high technology medicine. It is somewhat confusing to lump these two problems together only for the reason that both are expensive. Catastrophic acute care can be an add-on to basic insurance protection; long-term care insurance requires its own special design.

The Requirements of Insurance—The distribution of long-term care costs is ideal for insurance. Any particular individual faces a relatively small probability of needing a large amount of long-term care, but for the few who do, it can be very expensive indeed. A 65-year-old today faces a 40 to 50 percent chance of being in a nursing home before he or she dies, but most of these stays will be brief and will not involve large expense. One-third to one-half of all admissions will be for less than three months (Cohen et al., 1986). Only a small proportion of the elderly, about 10 percent, stay in nursing homes over a year, but it is this group that uses 90 percent of nursing home resources. The total nursing home costs, on average, for persons who stay for 1 year or longer is estimated to be about $100,000 (Commission on College Retirement, 1986).

Given these facts, individual saving is not an efficient means of meeting the cost of long-term care. If each individual saves to meet a high cost that will be experienced by only a few, the majority, for no good reason, will have cut back on the use of their money for other purposes. However, if each individual contributes the relatively small cost of average use, the group as a whole can be insured for a relatively low premium.

But there is more than the distribution of cost to deciding whether the application of insurance to a given risk is appropriate. Individual voluntary insurance, in particular, involves many other issues. First, will the individual be able to self-select coverage in a way that results in insuring a disproportionate number of those most likely to incur the risk (adverse selection)? Second, will the occurrence of the risk insured against be subject to the control of the insured? Third, can the risk be precisely enough defined so that valid claims can be paid and invalid ones denied? Fourth, how much will the use of a service increase as a result of its cost being reduced or eliminated by the insurance plan (induced costs)? Finally, the plan has to be administrable at a reasonable cost.

Uncertainty in any of these areas makes insurers understandably wary. As a result, private insurers have not marketed long-term care insurance agressively. The policies that are offered tend to cover only nursing home care, because the costs are easier to predict than the costs of home care. They pay indemnity amounts of a fixed number of dollars per day, thus avoiding both the problem of varying prices among nursing homes and the difficult problem of protection against inflation. The policies also limit the length of time for which payment will be made and usually try to screen out those with prior conditions that make them likely to need nursing home care in the near future.

These limiting conditions are certainly not a result of private insurers being unmindful of the needs of the elderly. However, to remain in business they have to safeguard against adverse selection, be reasonably sure that the individual is not in a position to create claims, limit liability to risks that can be measured and be able to estimate the "moral hazard" of increasing utilization resulting from the fact of the insurance itself. Thus the industry has been correctly cautious in selling individual voluntary insurance for long-term care. The result is very little coverage indeed—between 400,000 and 500,000 policies altogether (U.S. Social Security Administration, 1987). The big companies are just now beginning to explore group insurance tied to the place of employment, a type of policy that avoids some, but by no means all, of the problems of individual voluntary insurance.

It remains to be seen whether private group insurance for long-term care will sell. Employers are greatly concerned about the cost of supplements to Medicare (mostly acute care), which they are already committed to pay, and seem more interested in cutting back than expanding. The unions have not pressed for this type of group coverage, which is largely useful to members who have been retired for a long time. For both these reasons employer-paid-for insurance modeled on that for acute care coverage is unlikely to be widespread.

It is more likely that employers will be willing to be the marketing and administrative mechanism for voluntary employee-paid-for protection along the lines being promoted by Travelers and some other insurance companies.

One problem common to all long-term care insurance that covers home care as well as nursing home care is the difficulty of administration. In the provision of acute care, both private and public insurance plans rely largely on the professional judgment of doctors as to what treatment is medically necessary and where it should be given—in the doctor's office or at a hospital, on an outpatient or inpatient basis. The insurance plan may influence treatment through

187

the establishment of standards and limits on what it will cover, but most of the decisions are determined according to the standard of generally accepted medical practice in the physician community. While subjective judgments are frequently involved, they are made by members of a highly trained and respected profession.

In long-term care insurance there is a different problem, which is not easily solved. In many cases, the proper determination of what long-term services are needed, for whom, and where they should be provided seems much more debatable, and there is no long-established profession to determine such questions. The administrator is no longer able to use "medical necessity" as a guide. Rather, the determination has to be based on an assessment of an individual's total situation—physical, mental and social—and what the patient and his or her family and friends can reasonably be expected to do to meet the need for long-term care on their own.

The determination of the site of care—whether home, community facility, or nursing home—must be worked out with the individual and the family. These functions have been performed by specially trained nurses, social workers, and other counselors in Medicaid and other programs already providing such care, but it would be unwise to minimize the increased difficulty of such a task in an insurance program based on the concepts of legally enforceable entitlement and equal treatment.

To make the decision that a person meets basic eligibility conditions such as the inability to perform three or more of the activities of daily living is probably no more difficult than a long-term total disability determination required for younger persons, as is now required by the disability insurance part of Social Security. It may not prove too troublesome, even, to assess the physical, mental, and social functioning of the individual. But it will take considerable skill to decide, in a way that is acceptable to the family and the individual, how much of the need for care can and should be met by family and friends, and to determine when care at home or in the community is less desirable than care in an institution. I believe it can be done under an insurance approach, but the task is formidable. Yet, there is no other way; the individual and the family can hardly be left to decide entirely on their own the quantity and timing of services to be provided at home or when a nursing home admission is most appropriate.

What Should Be Done?—I would like very much to support a solution to the problem of financing long-term care that is an equal partnership between a federal insurance program and private insurance. I believe the phrase "equal partnership" would have an immediate political appeal. The forces that could be organized behind such a formula would make it nearly irresistible. The notion, consequently, is very attractive. Candor, however, requires me to say that, as in Medicare, the partnership will need to be quite unequal, with the federal plan doing the major part of the job and private insurance playing the supplementary role of filling in gaps not covered by the basic plan.

If, as some have suggested, the federal plan were to provide protection only after a very long waiting period, say two years, with private insurance assigned the task of covering the first two years, the plan would be faced with the inequities described earlier in connection with a catastrophic plan based on a fixed dollar threshold. It would work for those who could afford private insurance and could be induced to buy it but leave uncovered for two years the great bulk of those who need protection. This is much too long a time for most people to be able to meet the cost on their own; Medicaid would still be the big payer.

The basic government plan will need to provide coverage without a significant waiting period. The role of private insurance should then be to sell supplementary protection to some of the relatively well-off who want to protect a legacy or who want to buy services not covered by the basic plan. There will be room for this kind of supplementation because the government plan should have a large coinsurance payment in the case of nursing home care, or perhaps a sizable user's fee. The object of the plan should be to reimburse only for expenses over and beyond room and board, as those costs should be met by regular retirement income; this calls for a sizable payment on the part of the insured. Some relatively well-off people may want to avoid making copayments for nursing home care as well as the smaller but still significant coinsurance that I believe should accompany long-term care provided in the home. Perhaps, too, private insurance can be sold to provide more amenities than the basic plan.

I hope we won't have to go through years of demonstrating the obvious—that private insurance cannot produce anything approaching adequate coverage and that the government will need to take the lead. Using very generous assumptions, the Brookings study on long-term care suggests, for example, that even by the year 2018, private insurance, at the most, might account for 12 percent of total nursing home expenditures (Rivlin, 1988). In making the simulations that led to this conclusion, the authors note that they deliberately made generous assumptions about the ability and willingness of the elderly to participate in such coverage (Wiener et al., 1987).

One reason that private group insurance will take so long to be even marginally effective is that insurers will find it very difficult to cover those already retired. Employers and unions are not likely to give a high priority to adding this kind of fringe benefit for those who left the company long ago. Employer-paid-for private group insurance will almost have to start with the idea of providing protection in the future for those still working. It would be possible, however, to encourage current workers to pay for insurance for their parents, as in the Travelers' approach, or to encourage retirees who can afford the high premiums to pay for their own protection, as in the Aetna plan for retired state employees in Alaska.

All this adds up to the possibility of some worthwhile private insurance being offered, but of a type and on a scale that taken alone would make only a small contribution to the protection needed by most people.

Social Insurance

Can social insurance do what private insurance cannot do on a sufficiently large scale? I believe so. Many, but not all, of the difficulties of private insurance are less formidable under social insurance. First, the system would be compulsory and universal, covering everyone who works, with a premium for those already retired. Consequently, adverse selection would not be a problem. Second, under social insurance the currently retired could be blanketed in as was done when Medicare started.

The plan should be a modest one; in some respects more modest, perhaps, than would sell well in the competitive market of private insurance. The costs should be kept low by helping only those who are very seriously disabled, and significant beneficiary payments should be required. A 30 percent copayment might be applied to nursing home costs, with a maximum reimbursement for these expenses. Supplemental Security Income should be made available for those who cannot make this payment out of Social Security, pension, and other current income and assets.

I believe that costs could be contained reasonably well under such a plan. There are natural safeguards against a big increase in nursing home utilization, and nursing home care is the most costly part of long-term care. Initially there will be some increase in utilization, since there are many people now who by any reasonable standard should be in nursing homes but for whom there is no room because of the strict state controls on nursing home expansion. However, partly compensating for this factor over time is the fact that cases similar to some of those now in nursing homes will be handled at home, assuming that reasonable support services become available. A user's fee or copayment that, on average, equals room and board costs would greatly reduce the economic incentive to enter a nursing home inappropriately. But even more important for utilization control, most individuals and their families look on admission to a nursing home with great reluctance and, except for short-term stays, as an alternative of last resort. Certainly older people themselves would seek out any reasonable alternative, and sons and daughters usually have strong feelings against forcing such a choice on their parents. It is true, on the other hand, that our use of institutions in the United States for the care of the disabled elderly is relatively low when compared with similar cultures that pay more of the cost—5 percent of all those over 65 in the United States, compared to about 7 percent in Canada and the United Kingdom.

On balance, I would not expect nursing home utilization rates by age and sex to grow very much under an insurance plan. Those who turn to nursing homes, I believe, would still be mostly the very disabled elderly, particularly those with dementia, or those without a spouse or other family members to help care for them at home. A modest increase might well be desirable. Certainly some families are going to extraordinary lengths and assuming unreasonable burdens to maintain disabled elderly people at home. At the same time, it seems to me that there are strong forces operating against the possibility of the plan causing the institutionalization of large numbers of older people who could be better cared for at home.

I anticipate that the problem of possible overuse will be largely in the area of home services. Consequently, home care should also have a sizable copayment to encourage careful usage of the services offered and to provide a continuing incentive for family and other informal care. This will be a difficult benefit to administer, and coverage should be phased in with expansion occurring only as experience warrants. It is essential, however, to have a home care alternative in place from the beginning. Nursing home care insurance alone could increase undesirable institutionalization and is certainly not in itself the solution that elderly persons and their families want.

191

Why Social Insurance?

But why propose a social insurance system instead of an improved means-tested program based on Medicaid principles? The answer is that the elderly and their families are not satisfied with a system that forces people into poverty before they can be helped. Welfare is not popular and insurance is—for good reasons.

The distinguishing characteristics of social insurance are that eligibility for benefits grows out of past earnings or contributions, with the benefits paid without a test of need. Thus, benefits are regarded as an earned right, without the stigma, uncertainty of financing, and lack of political support frequently associated with programs designed solely for those with low incomes. Moreover, since social insurance pays benefits without regard to other income and resources, the recipients can add savings and private insurance to their basic benefits.

Welfare, in contrast, is supported from general taxes, and the amount of benefit and eligibility depends on the income and resources of the family. There is no requirement of past service on contribution, only current need.

In insurance, applicants demonstrate that they have worked sufficiently to be eligible or have made contributions toward their protection. In relief and assistance, applicants demonstrate a lack; proving the absence of enough to get along on. If they have income and resources, they are required to use these first. Those who have been self-supporting throughout most of their lives dislike the prospect of being dependent on such a program almost as much as they dislike the prospect of being a burden to their children.

Thus, I believe there will be great interest in a program of social insurance for long-term care designed to prevent need rather than simply to deal with it after it occurs. This interest will be especially strong on the part of the middle-aged workers who are concerned about the possible long-term care needs of parents, as well as later for themselves. In a very real sense, a social insurance program designed to meet the cost of long-term care can be thought of as middle-aged people sharing the risk of having to provide for their parents' care. Under insurance, the high cost in money and service now falling on the few would be spread among the many.

Support for this type of protection will come not only from elderly people themselves but also from their sons and daughters. Thus the provision of long-term care insurance through the federal government could soon become a political issue with wide appeal. Under present arrangements, a high proportion of middle-aged people may well be faced with a poignant choice. They can either take an elderly parent into their own homes, without adequate support services and with consequent disruption of careers and the loss of time and money, or they can send the parent to a Medicaid nursing home, frequently against his or her wishes. A national system is very much needed which can ease some of the burden on the family through home care benefits or alternatively (together with regular retirement income and Supplemental Security Income if retirement income is insufficient) through nursing home care.

We need to proceed with the difficult job of designing an effective federal long-term care insurance program; there is simply no other good way to meet the growing costs and to organize the improved services that are needed. We have some time, but not much. I would guess that we might be faced with the need to implement a long-term care social insurance plan as early as 1992 or 1993. The timetable might be something like this: debate on the concept as an important issue in the 1988 campaign, development plans by the executive branch during 1989, congressional consideration in 1990, and an effective date possibly as early as 1992.

Developing a program to take care of, and finance, the catastrophic and long-term care needs of our nation is a task to which we should apply Abraham Lincoln's philosophy of positive government:

> The legitimate object of government is to do for a community of people whatever they need to have done but cannot do at all or cannot do so well for themselves in their separate and individual capacities.

References

Cohen, Marc A.; Eileen T. Tell; and Stanley S. Wallack. "The Lifetime Risks and Costs of Nursing Home Use Among the Elderly." *Medical Care Review* 4 (December 1986): 1166.

Commission on College Retirement. *A Plan to Create Comprehensive Group Long-Term Care Insurance for College and University Personnel.* New York: Commission on College Retirement, 1986, p. 10.

Freeman, Howard et al. "Americans' Report on their Access to Health Care." *Health Affairs* 1 (Spring 1987): 6–18.

Robert Wood Johnson Foundation: *Access to Health Care in the United States.* Special Foundation Survey No. 2. New York, NY: Robert Wood Johnson Foundation, 1987.

Rivlin, Alice, et al. *Caring for the Disabled Elderly: Who Will Pay?* Washington, DC: Brookings Institution, 1988.

U. S. Congress. House. Committee on Ways and Means. *Background Material and Data on Programs within the Jurisdiction of the Committee on Ways and Means.* Washington DC: U.S. Government Printing Office, 1987, table 12, p. 219.

U. S. Department of Health and Human Services. Social Security Administration. Task Force on Long-Term Health Care Policies. "Survey of Policies in Force." In *Report to Congress and the Secretary.* Washington, DC: Government Printing Office: 1987, pp. 72–74.

Wiener, Joshua M.; Ray Hanley; Denise Spence; and Sheila Murray. Testimony presented at a hearing on long-term care, Subcommittee on Health, Ways and Means Committee, U.S. House of Representatives, March 31, 1987, p. 17.

XV. A Question of Commitment

REMARKS OF KAREN IGNAGNI

Ms. IGNAGNI: You read the papers and then you realize the four well reasoned but different solutions that have been suggested confirm the old axiom that where you stand depends on where you sit. Listening to Robert Ball crystallized my thoughts—that where we are today in this debate is in a large measure attributable to where we have been in the access area.

I do not think we will solve the long-term care problem soon. I think it is going to be the 1990s before we solve it, but we are probably where people were in the late 1960s and early 1970s with respect to pre-ERISA thinking, and in the early 1960s with respect to pre-Medicare thinking.

Had we had this discussion several years ago, I do not think anyone would have suggested the option of a public sector solution. But as we think today about this option versus a more limited reinsurance function for the public sector, I would urge you to think about the Pension Benefit Guaranty Corporation (PBGC). That program's history offers a model for dealing with the long-term care problem.

This is not merely a current health problem. This is a long-term problem, for which we will have to prefund. We must view it like pension systems and begin to think in these terms. For example, under PBGC, certain employers can do very nicely with the reinsurance system, based on such factors as the nature of their work force, the age of their workers, and the risk of their industry. Other employers, given the economic context and the challenges that they face—LTV Corporation* and many others—do not do so well. There are parallels here with respect to the type of adverse selection that certain employers would face were they to take the long-term care problem on themselves.

Mixed Signals from the Federal Government

We are getting mixed signals from the federal government. On the one hand, the government is definitely cost shifting to the private

---

*Editor's note: The LTV Corporation's movement in 1986 to cease retiree health benefits on filing for Chapter 11 bankruptcy brought public outcry and prompted swift congressional action.

sector. On the other hand, Congress has taken away the tax breaks previously given to employers to prefund retiree health care benefits, and that is a major problem.

Millions of people between the age of 55 and 65, particularly in the basic manufacturing industries, have taken advantage of 55-and-out programs and do not have any protection whatsoever. Basic access is an issue we need to discuss. Employers are not a homogeneous group. Some are not providing any health care protection while others offer comprehensive benefits. Those in the latter group—and we bargain with them every day—are not in very good shape because they are now faced with increased premium costs (in the range of 18 to 20 percent), because medical care inflation is on the rise. So we factor in an additional burden with long-term care, which leads many people to talk about flexible benefits. Flexible benefits, some argue, would allow employees the option of financing long-term care themselves and taking their own deductions. From an efficiency standpoint, I do not see how there are any economies of scale working in that kind of system, or why the federal government should want to encourage it.

Getting Workers to Focus on the Long-Term Care Issue

Another issue is how we are going to get people to focus on long-term care issues and take them seriously. It is difficult to gain the attention of workers between age 30 and 40. The AFL-CIO's members, which are a varied group—construction, service, blue collar, white collar—perceive that they have other, more important responsibilities.

One group says, "Well, we are just having our first child between 30 and 40, so we have got all those expenditures to worry about." Another group says, "Well, we're worrying about college costs." And the group that does respond is, of course, the group that has an elderly mother or elderly father at home, a family member in a nursing home, or one who may go into a nursing home. So we have intergenerational conflicts with respect to how we handle this.

When you talk to young employees about health care benefits at bargaining tables, more often than not lately, they want to move away from comprehensive benefits because they say, "Well, we want day care, we want education, we want other kinds of things." Older employees are interested in comprehensive health care packages, which only exacerbates the adverse selection problem.

At the AFL-CIO we are trying to sort out these issues, look for the system that distributes the cost most effectively and is equitable in terms of future costs. This is leading to a system which approaches universality, whether it consists of buying insurance through pools at the state or regional level (because one employer dealing with one insurer does not make sense over the long haul) or buying through the Social Security system.

Problems of Employers "Going It Alone"

We do not believe that employers are going to solve this problem individually, nor do we encourage them to do so, because that would involve a kind of risk that would be quite difficult to deal with, not just at the bargaining table, but within the entire economy. An employer could never be sure whether other employers with whom he is competing are offering the same level of coverage. This is similar to the dilemma associated with the health care access issue—employer A provides coverage, employer B does not; employer B gets jobs and bids because it has lower labor costs owing to the fact that it does not provide coverage.

All these things have to be factored in. There are no easy solutions.

XVI. Part Four Discussion

Is Medicaid Part of the Problem or the Solution?

Ms. YOUNG: I wanted to ask Robert Ball why you are so concerned about access if you have a program in which private insurance paid for the first one, two, or three years or for the first $2,000. Under normal circumstances, what you are saying would be absolutely true, that you would have the problem of $2,000 not being very much for one person, but representing a lifetime's assets for another person. Under current circumstances, that person is already being covered by Medicaid and perhaps, as some have said doing better under Medicaid than people with lower middle-class income. Since people can spend-down if they have very few resources, or immediately go into a nursing home under Medicaid if they have no resources, why you see this as a problem?

MR. BALL: Medicaid is certainly a lot better than nothing, and I am not attacking the services provided by Medicaid in many states, but people generally do not like the idea of being dependent on a program that requires them to dispose of their assets and have very low income before they gain protection. That is the reason some insurance companies would like to sell a two-year policy and then have a government insurance program pick up from there. They know people do not like to be dependent on a program like Medicaid.

The problem is that I do not think they will be able to approach anything like adequate coverage during those first two years. Private insurance companies can sell such a policy, but they would sell it largely to relatively well-off people who want to protect their assets.

Fostering Public-Private Partnerships at the State Level

MR. SOMERS: The Robert Wood Johnson Foundation for some time has been listening to the debate over the gap between prospects for satisfactory, comprehensive private long-term care insurance coverage and the aspirations of some for a major federal level, long-term care insurance program. We feel that we have to look for opportunities to invest relatively limited venture capital in testing a variety of long-term care insurance products.

199

We have taken a modest step into this swampy territory between the purely private and the purely public response. We hope to foster public-private partnerships at the state level, and we have made two planning grants to the states of Massachusetts and Connecticut to pursue that purpose.

Our objective is to address the need for rationalizing a very unpredictable system for financing long-term care in this country. We hope that by doing so we can protect elderly individuals from "nursing home/home care roulette" and give them personal security in terms of their health care and their financial status.

We can certainly continue to debate back and forth whether a model can be designed that will protect both individuals' assets and their health care needs and also be equitable. I've heard enough of the debate to believe that it is, at least, worth examining plans aimed at accomplishing both.

The states are in the best position at this time to gather and analyze the data that would be needed by the public sector and private insurers in order to design adequate, affordable long-term care insurance products. Many states have access to invaluable Medicaid data, nursing home utilization data, and other information critical to the analytical process we need to undertake to advance this field of insurance.

The Foundation is also very concerned about the lack of infrastructure for long-term care services. The design and development of the infrastructure for managing long-term care is one of the principal objectives of the planning grants that we have given and that we hope to give. A great deal of work has already been done in this area in Connecticut and Massachusetts.

Finally, I believe that in terms of political support for the implementation of possible demonstration programs, which we also hope to help fund, it appears to be most appropriate to start working at the state level. The debate will and should certainly go on at the national level. And the ultimate solution to the long-term care financing problem may have to come from the federal government. In the interim, however, we believe it is well worth investing in public/private partnerships in states where governors' commissions or legislative actions have already committed the state to further steps.

Life Care at Home

There is another concept that we are very excited about in the long-term care financing area which has not been mentioned yet today.

That is life care at home, which is essentially the traditional life care concept without the residential community or the housing. When people can stay at home, they can buy into the lifetime guaranteed long-term care insurance plan at a much lower cost. The concept is being tested in the Philadelphia area with our assistance and we are considering three more sites across the country.

I would like to have a program during the first two years and afterwards that was generally available to most people and provided them with a sense of security.

MR. BALL: I do not want to be left in the un-American position of not seeming to favor any partnership between the public and private sectors. It is merely that I see private insurance having a relatively small role—about like Medicare and Medigap insurance.

Sources of Revenue for a Social Insurance Program

Ms. SPENCE: I would like Mr. Ball to expand a bit more on the sources of revenue for a social long-term care insurance program. You mentioned that it could be similar to financing the Social Security system?

MR. BALL: Yes. I like the payroll tax. I think it is a fine tax.

First of all, it is not correctly described as a payroll tax. It is a deduction from workers' earnings; that is an income tax by anybody's definition. It is not shifted anywhere, it is borne by the worker. Then the employer makes a matching contribution from the payroll. Workers don't have payrolls, employers do. So, it is a payroll tax as far as the employer is concerned.

It is shifted, probably mostly to the employee, and the result is similar to a user's tax. What is wrong with that? Everything does not have to be supported by a highly progessive tax.

Actually, I am worried about the present financing of Medicare Part A as perhaps being too progressive. A $40,000-a-year worker is paying four times as much for exactly the same benefits as a $10,000-a-year worker under the program. You want to make it more progressive? I think that a system of deductions from workers' earnings matched by employers' contributions is a really good way—and one used throughout the world—to support programs like this. Such financing reinforces the concept of a right to the benefit. I think contributions are a great idea.

Now, I would not only do that. You do have a big catch-up problem in this program—coverage of those already retired—and I like very

201

much the idea of a part of such cost being borne by an earmarked estate tax. I think there is a lot to be said for that idea, given who the beneficiaries are.

We have very largely destroyed the estate tax in the last few years. I would like to restore it. I am not a great fan of passing on large assets from one generation to the next; some, yes, but I think an estate tax would be a good way to finance part of the backlog.

Mr. Rother mentioned a few other finance sources that could well be considered. A health program has some basis for partial support from a tobacco and liquor tax. Now that we have the income tax in fairly good shape, surtaxes on the income tax, earmarked for specialized purposes are also a pretty good way of raising money for a program like this.

A major point to remember is that people in the United States are not aware of the fact that they are way undertaxed compared to most other industrialized countries. When you take into account state, local, and federal government taxes, and compare the total with the total taxes collected by other countries, you find that we do not do nearly as much through the public sector as all our major trading partners.

So, when businessmen say, "You put me at a terrible competitive disadvantage," the right question is: With whom? Germany? No. United Kingdom? No. Who? Not even Japan, now.

MR. SALISBURY: South Korea and Taiwan.

Tax Incentives to Encourage Private-Sector Initiatives

MS. BORZI: I wanted to make a couple of comments about the role of the federal government to encourage private-sector initiatives by providing tax incentives.

Several of the comments have alluded to the need to reverse the prefunding limitations imposed as a result of the changes made in the Deficit Reduction Act (DEFRA).

As a point of reference for those of you who do not know me, I am not a staff person from the tax committee. I work for the House Education and Labor Committee and, in 1984, the members of our committee, on a bipartisan basis, went on public record as having opposed as ill-advised the repeal of those tax incentives in DEFRA.

I have to make a personal confession here—I think that we made a mistake in advocating that those tax incentives should not be re-

202

pealed. I am publicly admitting this for the first time. I suppose I should have issued my usual disclaimer that this is my opinion only. It does not represent the opinions of the Committee on Education and Labor, the Subcommittee on Labor-Management Relations, or any of its members, particularly its chairman.

I have learned a lot in the three years since that June weekend in 1984 when I went to Hawaii to give a speech. Nothing was supposed to happen on DEFRA, but, of course, it did. So I came right back. I have learned a lot since then—not only not to go to Hawaii during consideration of a tax bill, but also that those good old days that I heard so many of you allude to today and have heard so many of you allude to in the past, were good old days only for employers.

They were not particularly good days for retirees or for participants in these plans. Everyone here has talked about the need of the employers to be able to prefund retiree health benefits, but no one has mentioned the lack of entitlement to those benefits.

What were employers prefunding? There was and continues to be a belief on the part of employers, except to the extent that the court so holds, that no formal entitlement, or a legal entitlement to any benefits whatsoever exists. It seems to me that the entitlement question is critical.

The idea that the federal government, whether we have a huge deficit or no deficit, simply is going to throw tax breaks willy nilly at anyone who has a great idea for funding some benefit is, I think, hopelessly naive.

A Clearer Definition of the Nature of the Promise

I think we need a vision to clarify what goals we are trying to achieve. Once it is clear that the private market, in partnership more or less with the federal government, is trying to reach these goals, they can be matched against proposed funding vehicles to determine whether they are worthy of tax-favored treatment.

Until we have a clearer definition of what the nature of the promise is, and the employer's liability to provide that promise, Congress is not going to provide tax breaks for prefunding retiree health or for prefunding long-term care policies, no matter how worthy we and many of the members of the Congress think those social objectives are.

What Is the Employer Liability?

Until we know where we are going, Congress is not going to say, "Go ahead, insurance companies, we will give you all these tax breaks to develop products you can market—but you decide to whom and to what end." I don't believe Congress will act until the important questions are answered: what is the legal entitlement under these policies, what is the nature of the promise, and what is employer liability? Once we know what the promise is, once we know what the employer liability is, then collectively we can figure out how to fund that promise, or determine if that promise needs to be funded at all.

I think the nature of the funding that is going to be required (whether it is prefunding, pay-as-you-go funding, or some variant of terminal funding) is going to be a function of what that liability is. Until these important questions are answered, you are deluding yourselves if you think that Congress, whether we have a budget deficit or not, will create new tax incentives to provide benefits of ambiguous design as a method of "dealing" with the "problem," when neither the problem nor the solution has been defined.

On the other hand, when that discussion takes place, I think you will find Congress willing to put its money where its mouth is. You will find both a substantial commitment of public funds and a willingness to help encourage private-sector initiatives in terms of tax incentives. But until that time, I don't think you're going to find Congress willing to do that, even if it had the means to do it—and reasonable people can differ as to whether it does or not.

The Need for Advance Funding

MR. GARBER: First, and what troubles me most about the whole public approach suggested, is that we would be introducing another plan that should be funded in advance and that will not be. The whole question of capital accumulation in this country would again get lost because we would be stepping up to pay something out of current income that should be funded.

I would be very disturbed if we were to take a Social Security approach to this and not seek to fund some of it in advance. I think this is a critical issue. We can hardly do too much advance funding. It would appear that much of the turmoil in the markets is due to our dependence on foreign investors; they have a considerable impact on the market, and we march to their tune to a considerable degree. If we continue down a road which does not call for funding benefits that should be funded in advance, we deserve what will happen to us.

Secondly, I have a considerable question about the degree to which this can be an employer-provided benefit. It seems to me that the problem with health benefits, unlike pensions, is that when an employee retires from a company, he or she usually receives the full set of postretirement health benefits that are provided to all of the company's retirees, regardless of whether they worked there 5 years or 50 years. Pension benefits have always recognized the amount of time that a person works in a company and have given them proportional benefits, but health benefits are difficult to limit in a similar manner and this is usually not done.

I think that this creates a considerable problem today in the area of retiree health benefits, a problem which would be exacerbated in the case of long-term care benefits. I believe this is the cause of the entitlement question raised by Phyllis Borzi. A major reason why companies are reluctant to provide an entitlement to such benefits is that they have no way of proportioning them appropriately.

If the benefit is to be largely or entirely employee-funded, the essential questions are affordability and portability. In these cases, what you really have then is an employer-sponsored plan, which is employee-funded and where the entitlements to those funds go with the employee.

Saving Money for a Benefit That May Never Be Paid

This brings me to my third point, and one that I have found troubling in all of this discussion. If, over my lifetime, I save a lot of money for long-term care benefits, I really do not want that money to go to somebody else. It is my money; I saved it, and I would rather spend it in my own way.

I think it would be hard to sell the concept of having insurance that is funded over a long term, that may never pay any benefits to me, and that has no cash value associated with it that I could take out if, at the age of 85, I decide I am never going to need the funds for long-term care. The insureds will feel that if they put their money into it and don't need to use it for long-term care, they ought to be able to use it as they want to use it because it is their money. I think that this attitude will create a problem in trying to market this insurance as an insurable-type benefit of the form usually described. It is a dilemma which I will leave you with.

MR. KITTREDGE: I can understand a person not wanting to turn over what is left over to someone else, but I think you have to recognize that the cost of funding long-term care coverage on your own would be far greater—perhaps four, five, six times as much—as the cost of insurance.

Increasing Longevity and Higher Long-Term Care Costs

MR VLADECK: Peter Libassi said something that raises another very basic point that we are in danger of overlooking. That is that one of the reasons we are facing a financial crisis for Medicaid programs and families with long-term care needs is because we have done such a good job of preventing premature mortality among the elderly over the last 20 or 25 years, at least to some extent because of the success of the Medicare program. The problem with prevention is that it ends up costing you a lot of money. I am not arguing against it, but I am arguing it is an illusion that there is a panacea out there if we get the 55-year-olds, like the 25-year-olds, to quit smoking.

The fact of the matter is that it is increasing longevity that is causing us a lot of these problems. It is of some worry to me that, despite the very dramatic gains in longevity at age 65 that we have seen since the advent of Medicare, most of the numbers I have seen pertaining to long-term care use and expenditures assume, at best, current life expectancies when there is reason to believe we will continue to do substantially better.

One of the problems we have always had with life care is that if you do too good a job taking care of people in life care communities or any other community care programs, they live longer than was predicted and they defy your actuarial assumptions.

This is a serious issue in terms of financing issues, and I do not want to treat it lightly. If you're going to keep people alive, it is going to cost you money. I think that is probably worth it.

Preventing Alzheimer's Disease

If we had a limited pot of money to use for long-term care, my first priority would be to prevent Alzheimer's disease because that is clearly the most cost-effective investment that a society could make. The benefit of prevention can be realized only with a much greater public commitment to biomedical research in this area. My second priority would be to provide greater community support for families who are providing the bulk of care.

The final point I wanted to raise is the fuzziness of what constitutes long-term care, because the amount of long-term care that is being provided today under the hospital system and paid for in the acute care system is phenomenal. I am not sure it is inappropriately placed care, but the point is we are already paying for it.

Better Managed Care

I wanted to ask either Tom O'Brien or John McCormack whether there has been any attempt to look seriously at what employers are already paying today for long-term care that is perhaps mislabeled and either categorized as disability or extended leave, or perhaps managed through acute care coverage when it could be more effectively managed in long-term care.

It seems to me that a very sizable financial stake already exists, and it needs to be better managed, regardless of whether or not you institute a new benefit. But I am not sure anyone has really looked at it that way.

MR. McCORMACK: We have looked at it from the standpoint of coordination with the medical program that does provide a degree of long-term health care as well as nursing home care, but not to the same extent as what we are proposing to add on.

The disability issue is a tough one. We have looked at it, but only in terms of our own internal experience, which is not necessarily universally applicable. But, yes, there is a series of benefits currently associated with long-term care that have to be better coordinated than they are. That is one of the reasons I mentioned that continuum of care, the concept of case management.

MR. O'BRIEN: We have looked hard at the social HMO (health maintenance organization) or the managed care options, and really favor them. But there are the problems with the federal government and getting HCFA (Health Care Financing Administration) approval for capitation. Also, many of the HMO's are now backing out of Medicare because it is too much trouble. They feel that they are getting squeezed and that they are going to lose out. However, the estimates are that the savings from managed care would pay at least half of the cost of long-term care.

A Coverage Problem for the Older Unemployed?

MR. CARTWRIGHT: I am with the National Institute on Aging, and I am a researcher in the economics of aging, and look forward to the conquest of Alzheimer's disease, which I have spent some time working on.

I have a question regarding the partnership and the roles of the private and public sectors. One of the interesting things about labor markets is that males who are 55 and over tend not to have such a great attachment to the labor market and, indeed, about 30 percent of that age cohort between 55 and 65 may not be working at all. They may be covered under their employee benefit plans for long-term care, but now when I'm 55, I'm declared superfluous and I lose my job—

MR. SALISBURY: I would only underline that there are some between those ages who willingly and by self-selection choose to define themselves as such. A great deal of that retirement is voluntary.

MR. CARTWRIGHT: A lot of it is also related to one's health because those who are not in the labor market are known to be less healthy than the 70 percent who have continued in the labor market. Whether or not it is voluntary or involuntary, health-related or not, is difficult to know. But regardless, how are these people going to continue their long-term care policies under these private plans? Are they just going to be thrown out? You can continue to pay for this on your own or not, or is the firm or the corporation going to continue making a contribution as part of the severance package? What is the answer to that?

MR. McCORMACK: The answer from our vantage point is the converted policy that would give the individual the opportunity to continue coverage without evidence of insurability. That is almost essential, I think. Once you provide the product, you just beg the issue of what happens upon termination if it is not a widespread benefit.

MR. SALISBURY: Both Margaret Gagliardi with American Express and Gail Schaeffer with John Hancock mentioned that their policies were being offered to current retirees and would also provide transitional coverage for those close to retirement. To the degree they are being designed, they are attempting to accommodate those employees.

MR. CARTWRIGHT: I see, though, that in the future it would tend to be an employee benefit arrangement.

MR. LIFSON: For many of those employees, the employer does, in fact, continue health benefits until they are first eligible for Medicare. So, there is no reason to believe that, if long-term coverage became an employee benefit, those same employers would not continue the benefit as they continue other benefits.

MR. WYSZEWIANSKI: I just want to share two reactions I have had in listening to this group. I had the interesting experience of working on a project on catastrophic health care costs that started in 1980, when the National Center for Health Services Research, through some incredible foresight, decided to award a contract for research on catastrophic insurance.

At that time it was perfectly acceptable to say that when we talk about catastrophic insurance, we are really talking about acute care. Even after President Reagan talked about catastrophic insurance, the first reaction was to go back to proposals like Senator Long's and see it as involving acute care only.* So several of us started saying, "Well, what about long-term care? That's a big source of the problem."

Now it seems that everybody has gotten religion, and we are here supposedly talking about catastrophic care but, except for the last two speakers, everyone is talking about long-term care. I am afraid we may be over-correcting. We forget the 50 million people out there who, by any reasonable definition, are at very great risk of having catastrophic expenditures. That is one reaction.

The other reaction is that since there is no one else here to defend them, I will stand up, as best I can, for physicians, HMOs and others, who would probably have something to say about the enthusiasm that one sometimes hears here for pluralism and letting all kinds of different programs develop.

Problems for the Providers

There are a great many providers out there—HMOs, hospitals, and so on—who are getting very tired of having 25 different payment plans, each requiring different documentation of quality and of the amount spent on certain procedures, different verification plans, different utilization programs, and so forth. These providers would rather

---

*Editor's note: The Long-Ribicoff catastrophic insurance bill of 1979 would have provided coverage to everyone whose out-of-pocket health care expenditures were greater than $2,000 (in 1979 dollars) during a year's time.

deal with one uniform, good or bad, but at least uniform, set of requirements and standards. I think that when we talk about pluralism and diversity we should consider that there may be a revolution brewing on the part of the health care providers who ultimately have to do all these things.

MR. JACKSON: In the pension field, having watched ERISA with joint and survivor requirements, MPPAA (Multiemployer Pension Plan Amendments Act) with withdrawal liability, REACT (1984 Retirement Equity Act) with surviving spouse benefits and qualified domestic relations orders, and group health COBRA (Consolidated Omnibus Budget Reconciliation Act of 1985) extension requirements, the last thing in the world the private sector needs is more government benefit design.

This is an area where the government tax rules, as they now stand, are draconian. If a company were to put money in a fund, and the fund were taxed as a corporation so that there is no tax break, the government now says, "Well, we have to tax somebody, so we'll tax the employees." I think you could set something up which is taxed as a corporation on the investment return but where the funds are kept away from the corporation itself, separate and not subject to the claims of creditors. That, to me, is not a tax break.

The basic attitude of the tax-writing committees is that every penny that a person earns belongs to the federal government if they don't take it, so we are lucky to have what we've got, I guess.

The second comment concerns Robert Ball's message. During the entire discussion of this new program that the federal government should get into in 1990 or 1992, I did not hear a single word about the status of the Medicare program which, on the basis of cost projections, is probably going to bankrupt America in the long run.

Medicare has been changed already to the point where some liabilities have been tossed back onto the private sector. More is expected in the future because Medicare financing just is not going to hold up. And the thought of taking on something else—amorphous, undesigned, no experience, and so on—is typical of the federal government. We will adopt it at a 2 percent tax. The tax will be 10 percent 10 years out, and 30 percent 20 years out, but how you raise the taxes to cover it will be somebody else's legislative concern.

MR. BALL: I wanted first to respond to the earlier thought that somehow Medicare was going to bankrupt the country. That seems unlikely in view of the fact that, almost without exception, all the major industrial countries not only have policies similar to Medicare

210

but do much more in their health care systems, and do it through the government, yet they do not seem to be on the verge of bankruptcy. They have been doing it for a long time, and many of them have an older population.

Insofar as there is anything to the point, I think it argues that our methods of reimbursement in the Medicare program have not been tough enough. It is not that the benefits are extraordinary. And that could be true in long-term care, unless we are very careful about both utilization and how we pay providers.

I don't think it is fair to the Congress or the Executive Branch to talk as if they have made changes in social insurance and imposed a small tax for the short term without looking at the long-range cost.

I think I have been in on every final conference on Social Security between the House and the Senate, from the mid-1940s until 1972. I know of no time when they were not focused at the end on the long-term costs.

People say that members of Congress have a horizon of about two years. In Social Security, they have the unbelievable horizon of 75 years. I can't believe it. The big issue in the 1983 legislation on the House floor—in fact, the only issue of any significance—was over a provision that didn't begin to take effect until the year 2000: the raising of the age of first eligibility for full benefits.

Congress has been extraordinarily responsible in legislating on social insurance programs. That is one of the reasons that leads me to prefer social insurance solutions. When you have earmarked taxes supporting future benefits, you are required to make long-term projections.

If you want to worry about financing government, worry about projecting defense expenditures, or worry about projecting any expenditures out of general revenue. Social insurance expenditures are carefully watched, and changes are made if things seem to be going wrong.

How far out do private health insurers project their costs? Two or three years? Not usually much further. I just do not think that was a fair criticism of government insurance. That is not a correct criticism of the way the Congress has behaved.

The Employer Defines the Promise

MS. BORZI: I wanted to reassure Paul Jackson that I was not talking about a federally designed package. I was talking about a system in which the employer decides the nature of the promise and communicates that promise, and then the nature of the promise is matched up with the liability. The simple example is that if the employer decides that the entitling event to this benefit is actual retirement from the company, you would fund something where the date of entitlement was retirement and not before. This is different from an approach such as FASB appears to be taking, which is to assume that these benefits accrued over the working life.

If you believe that you can terminate your plan today and have no continuing liability to anybody under the plan, then there is no reason to provide advance funding of that benefit, because there is no benefit to be funded after the plan terminates.

The employer defines the promise, and then its funding ability is a function of what the promise is and how long it extends.

MR. SALISBURY: I assume that what Mr. Jackson is referring to is the intermediate actuarial assumptions from the Medicare trustees report, which indicate that to support the current benefit program the Medicare payroll tax would have to eventually rise to cover 7 percent from the current rate of less than 3 percent. This would be a very significant increase in the tax burden. Whether it is too much or too little is a wholly different issue.

MR. SALISBURY: Frank McArdle, EBRI's director of Education and Communications has participated in a couple of different international sessions in the last two years, where many of those foreign governments that tax much more heavily and provide much more in the way of benefits are currently wrestling with the potential necessity of cutting back those programs, of attempting to find private alternatives to supplement them. They do not believe that they are going to be able to continue to afford what they are now providing.

So, I think the affordability issue vis-à-vis all of the system is still a realistic issue and concern.

Actuarial and Legal Liability

MR. HARRINGTON: We put into effect a program in which we projected future postretirement death benefits and we funded them. I believe that there is an actuarial liability there, but it does not mean that all of the liability is fully vested now. We put up the money because we believe over time these benefits will become payable and earnings on reserve assets will offset the adverse economic consequences of a rising incidence of expense to the corporation while at the same time securing the benefit to the employee. DEFRA has hit

212

us right between the eyes, after having set up that funding mechanism.

With respect to prior comments, we have measured the retiree life liability for death benefits and we have certainly projected such figures for at least 75 years. So, I think the private plans fully reflect the cost of such benefits.

The bottom line is that plan sponsors do look at the implications of their programs; they look at the actuarial liability and the rate at which such liability is emerging; they look at the impact on their product line, and finally at the implications of the intergenerational transfer of expenses. If you are trying to sell a product over the working lifetime of employees and if you do not fund the benefits or if you do not budget for them properly, you have an unyielding increase in charges to expense resulting from benefits to your retirees. The costs are there, and the projections reflect them.

We can't pull the medical now. You cannot even start to recognize that liability even though you are going to be in it because you can get hung up on vesting. Many of us believe—and many attorneys would argue—that you have cases of applied contract, and that is where the courts are coming out.

Ms. BORZI: My point is exactly that. If the legal liability is to provide a benefit for life, then you should have an opportunity to prefund that benefit because you have a legal obligation. If the unscientific survey of the number of people who come through my doorway and sit on my couch is any representation, I would say that 99 percent say this: "I am an employer. I want to continue the plan permanently." Some even go so far as to say: "I believe I have a moral obligation to continue the plan permanently but, as a bottom line, I do not have a legal obligation."

If people do not have a legal obligation, then I do not think it is appropriate to let them prefund for a liability that they do not have. If they do have a legal obligation, then I think Congress would be willing to let people prefund to the extent necessary to meet that liability.

The Private Sector as a Generator of Ideas and Innovation

MR. LIBASSI: Over the last five years, we have seen a major change in the private sector on this issue of long-term care, and we have seen a rapid evolution of policies. We have already heard hints that we may be moving from insurance to other mechanisms in the private sector, whether it is pension or savings or some other conversion strategy that will enable the private sector to meet these needs. While I certainly do not want to suggest that the government does not have a major role, I think we should not prematurely discard that very powerful engine in our society—the private employer sector—to generate ideas, to create new products, and to find new ways to meet multiple responsibilities.

PART FIVE
WHAT DOES THE FUTURE HOLD?

The papers and discussion in the earlier chapters of this book have explored definitions of catastrophic and long-term care costs and the implications of those definitions for public and private policy. Millions of Americans face such expenses, either because they lack health insurance coverage or because their coverage is inadequate. Government programs such as Medicare and Medicaid and employer-sponsored health plans all provide coverage—but gaps exist. And for many, the elderly in particular, the truly catastrophic health care expense is long-term care in a nursing home. In the concluding chapters of *Where Coverage Ends: Catastrophic Illness and Long-Term Health Care Costs* the authors try to predict what the future holds for the issues of catastrophic and long-term care.

Steven A. Grossman looks at these issues from the perspective of what he calls five "controlling facts" associated with long-term care (chapter XVII). (1) The number of persons most likely to need long-term care is large and growing. (2) Future costs of providing long-term care services are enormous. (3) Federal and state governments account for almost half of national nursing home expenditures. (4) Long-term care is fundamentally different from acute care because it encompasses services and needs that are both medical and social. (5) Long-term care is not inherently catastrophic.

Grossman says that these points lead him to conclude that there is an urgency in setting up financing mechanisms and building up reserves to cover the costs of long-term care. He also contends that long-term care is too costly for a significant expansion in the public sector, although government will continue to play a major role. Finally, financing options must be carefully designed to preserve choices and flexibility and to encourage individual and family responsibility.

In chapter XVIII, Bruce Vladeck cautions that an emphasis on long-term care problems should not lead to the exclusion of a focus on the millions of Americans without health insurance, including millions of uninsured children. He also sees an anomaly in talk of developing a new broad-scale benefit to cover long-term care while other benefits, particularly ones provided by employers, are being reduced.

Vladeck argues that one way to expand coverage for the uninsured population would be to destigmatize Medicaid and partially subsidize care from the private sector. He also discusses integrating the Medicare program as it now exists with a future long-term care program and developing service delivery systems for long-term care under Medicare.

Vladeck states that the existing Medicare system increases costs and causes difficulties for beneficiaries by creating barriers between it and other financing systems. The situation is particularly acute, he says, in terms of home care. Vladeck also describes what he calls a crisis in the home care field relating to quality of service and a lack of standards.

Catastrophic expense has to be measured, says Edward F. Howard, in terms of its impact on the people for whom it is a catastrophe (chapter XIX). He lists costs that do not show up, particularly in home care bills, such as the disruption in the lives and careers of the families who take care of a chronically ill relative.

Howard predicts that there will be standards set for long-term care and that there will be a public role in setting those standards. He believes that private insurance faces many hurdles in dealing with such factors as adverse selection and the long period between the time individuals pay for benefits and the time they receive them. Howard concludes that low- and moderate-income elders have the greatest stake in the long-term care debate, and he suggests that private insurance will not be developed to meet that need.

The Part Five discussion in chapter XX focuses on the home health care option and its cost and practicality in relation to nursing home care.

216

XVII. Building Reserves and Preserving Flexibility for Long-Term Care

REMARKS OF STEVEN A. GROSSMAN

Most individuals familiar with long-term care know myriad facts and figures that may be useful in understanding the complexities of long-term care financing. However, based on the work the U.S. Department of Health and Human Services (HHS) has done, I would argue that a relatively small number of facts and figures control the dynamics of the future and define the parameters of possible solutions.

I would like to highlight what I consider the top five controlling facts about long-term care and explain where these facts take us. I will make predictions about what I think the future holds. However, let me give advance warning that none of my predictions provides any neat solution to the problems before us.

Growing Numbers in Need of Long-Term Care

Fact one. The number of persons most likely to need long-term care is large and growing. The number of elderly persons is going to increase from 11 percent of the population—28 million people—in 1984 to 21 percent of the population—65 million persons—by the year 2030. The number of persons over age 85, those most likely to need long-term care services, will increase three to four times as fast as the general population during the same period. If you are age 85 or older, we already know that you are four times more likely to spend time in a nursing home, and fifteen times more likely to need assistance with personal care.

Clearly, more people are going to need long-term care in the next 40 to 50 years. Virtually every year, the number will increase, and it will become enormous compared to what it is today.

Enormous Future Costs

Fact two. Even conservative estimates of the future costs of providing long-term care services are huge. In 1985, the nation spent roughly $38 billion on long-term care services for persons of all ages, including $26 billion for nursing home care for the elderly. By the year 2020, costs for nursing home care alone are expected to exceed

$100 billion, *in 1987 dollars.* As the population ages, and the number of people in the over 65 cohort increases, health costs to the nation will nearly triple. Added to this is the effect of inflation, which in the nursing home industry has for years far exceeded inflation in the rest of the economy.

Any extensive long-term care financing system, whether public or private, will also induce a certain amount of additional demand for services and raise overall costs if it replaces out-of-pocket expenditures. The amount of increase in costs is speculative.

In the long-term care section of the report, *Catastrophic Illness Expenses*, that HHS Secretary Otis Bowen sent to the President in 1986, we projected induced demand at between 11 and 38 percent, depending on the type of financing options and associated out-of-pocket costs. That would be the increase in demand over and above the current level of services projected forward and adjusted for demographics. I understand that when Medicare came into being, the number was more like 100 percent above projections, so we think 11 to 38 percent is conservative.

Many of the projections you will see for long-term costs do not add on any factor for induced demand. But our report stressed that when you project out over a number of years a factor of increased demand, it adds up to substantial additional dollars.

Thus, my second fact is that, wherever the money comes from, the cost of long-term care will be high.

State and Federal Government Commitment

Fact three. Federal and state government funds already account for almost one-half of the nation's nursing home care expenditures. This is a level of effort not far off the present public sector contribution toward acute-care cost for the elderly. There are major differences, however, in how the balance of expenditures are paid. Forty-nine percent of nursing home care is paid directly out-of-pocket, and private insurance pays less than 1 percent.

The point is that we are not talking about a question of whether or not public funds will play a major role. They do now. There is absolutely no indication from any source I have of any attempt to cut that back. Through Medicaid and other programs, federal, state, and local governments will be at least a 50-50 partner in the foreseeable future.

The real issue for the future is how the remaining 50 percent will be financed. How do we best rationalize this expense in order to serve peoples' needs at a reasonable cost to society?

So, the third fact is that there is already a government-state involvement that amounts to a full partnership with the private sector.

Differences between Acute and Long-Term Care

Fact four. Long-term care is fundamentally different from acute care. Long-term care encompasses services and needs that are both medical and social in nature. Unlike acute health care, for example, which often depends on services delivered by highly skilled professionals, long-term care involves people and services that can be delivered by you and me. In fact, the largest portion of long-term care in this country is, indeed, delivered by family members, individuals who are not highly skilled health care professionals.

Further distinguishing long-term from acute care is the fact that people needing long-term care often have alternatives in the form of various combinations of services and living arrangements that can be packaged to serve their particular need. A person needing his or her appendix out has relatively little choice compared to the options available in long-term care.

The need for long-term care services is also highly variable and is related not only to a patient's condition but also to his or her living arrangements, the availability of family and friends, the availability of community services, and many other nonmedical factors. Some of this variability is inherent in long-term care. It is evidenced in the often-quoted point that for every person living in a nursing home there are an estimated two others with similar disabilities and care needs living in the community. In other words, by looking only at peoples' physical state you cannot account for why one individual is in a nursing home while two others in similar condition are not.

All these factors make it difficult to predict or regulate the kinds of services that will be needed and when they will be needed, particularly those such as home care, that do not involve a nursing home.

In summary, the fourth controlling fact is that long-term care and acute care are different. We need to acknowledge this difference, or we may devise solutions that will be unsatisfactory and may be unduly expensive.

Long-Term Care Not Inherently Catastrophic

Fact five. Long-term care is not inherently catastrophic in a financial sense. It is often taken for granted that catastrophic and long-term care expenses are synonymous. However, the great majority of disabled older persons who live in the community (about 4.6 million individuals) remain in their own homes and receive most of the care they need from family and friends, at little or no *direct financial* cost to themselves or to the public.

Because of the strength of this informal care system, catastrophic home care expenses for this group are relatively rare. Estimates based on HHS's 1982 long-term care survey indicate that of the 4.6 million disabled older persons living in the community, fewer than 600,000 persons paid for any formal home care services with out-of-pocket funds; and a similar number received some formal (paid) care provided at no cost to them but at a cost to someone else (e.g., government, voluntary agency, and so forth).

Median expenses for those who did purchase some formal home care services were about $40 a month, and the average expenses were $164 per month. Only a very small segment—60,000 persons—incurred very large home care expenses of $400 a month and more. The majority of older persons who need long-term care receive it at home, from family, at very little cost, certainly not in the catastrophic range.

I acknowledge that these figures do not take into account acute-care expenses or other emergencies which can drain the financial resources of the elderly. Nor do they reflect the emotional strain or sacrifices of time and effort that is often necessary to keep disabled persons at home. They simply indicate that for the majority, the immediate and direct financial costs of long-term care are modest.

Funding Rapid Increases in Costs

What do these five facts that I have recounted suggest? First, it seems to me that the problem is urgent. We probably have a fairly short window to set up financing mechanisms and, most importantly, to begin building up reserves, whether we pursue private or public mechanisms.

If we, as a society, do not begin building up a reserve of funds to pay benefits, we will be in the position of trying to fund rapid increases in the cost of long-term care services out of current income. This is what we have done with Social Security.

220

I would also note that we are seeing some of the same problems with companies that could not afford to prefund their retiree health benefits. We need to consider long-term care in terms of prefunding. We need to have the will and commitment to prefund benefits.

Second, the government already pays half the costs and thus already plays a major role. I think we should seek to broaden the financial base to other payers, not consolidate it on the backs of taxpayers through additional taxes.

Designing Financing Options

Third, the diversity of needs, the circumstances of long-term care, and the importance of informal care provided by families suggest that the financing options we adopt must be carefully designed to preserve choices and flexibility as well as to encourage individual and family responsibility.

The facts suggest that to the extent that we intend to shield families against catastrophic expenses, as a priority, public money should be spent on base coverage for nursing home services rather than for home care. Home care is a moral good—there are many noneconomic reasons to support it. It is a humane option. It keeps people independent. However, in most cases, expenses associated with home care do not seem to be a determining factor in decisions about whether or not a person needs to go to a nursing home.

Traditional Responsibility of Government

Finally, the facts suggest that in today's economic climate, long-term care is too costly for a significant expansion in the public sector, the federal government in particular.

Let me be clear, however, how I view the public sector role. No one is suggesting that the federal and state governments retrench and pay less. I think the overall question is, should we pay more from public funds? There are several subsets of this question.

Should we pay more before we try to develop private financing alternatives that can mitigate the impact of long-term care costs for individuals? Should we pay more out of public funds for people who can afford to protect themselves by purchasing long-term care insurance? Should we pay more for people who want to pass on their estates relatively intact to their children? In short, should we pay more for people who can afford to pay for their own care?

221

Most of the thinking right now in regard to a public system inevitably has us paying significant amounts of money to provide protection for people who would not normally come to the public rolls because they would find resources or alternatives outside the public sector.

In my view, the government's policy in financing long-term care should focus on the traditional responsibility of government: should we pay more for those persons who have no private resources, and should we pay more for those who, despite advance planning and family resources, encounter long-term care costs well beyond ordinary means?

In February 1987, President Reagan asked the Treasury Department to study the tax implications of a number of recommendations from the Department of Health and Human Services that were designed to encourage personal savings for long-term care and the purchase of long-term care insurance.

We have been working with Treasury staff and expect a report shortly. In the meantime, the department is working on public-private sector initiatives to increase consumer awareness of the need for better protection. We are also working with researchers, insurance companies, and actuaries to improve the data on long-term care needs and financing.

To close, I will hazard two predictions. First, I predict that a fully public sector comprehensive solution will not be enacted anytime over the next several years. I think the economic climate and the budget deficit, combined with the high cost, make a fully public-sector approach too difficult to manage in terms of a concrete proposal.

I have, for instance, seen the results of the Villers-AARP survey, which indicate that many people want this benefit and are willing to pay for it. I would suggest, however, that the poll results did not consider the potential for sticker-shock—when taxpayers are confronted with real numbers, the willingness to pay may be very different. I think we can afford to get started in other ways—other than, say, for the federal government to do it all.

My second prediction is that private sector initiatives will develop very fast. One can see that private options, insurance particularly, are only just getting started. American Express and John Hancock already have group insurance offerings to employees under development and other companies are ready to follow.

My concern here, along with my prediction that the private-sector role will grow, is that the full effect of private-sector initiatives will be muted if the public rhetoric is so determinedly anti-private sector that insurance companies feel the market will be taken away. We must give companies room to work and to make inroads into a market which I believe exists. I know there is a lot of talk that only the wealthy can afford long-term care insurance, but I do not think that the numbers totally bear that out.

Our own study did some economic modeling. For example, if you use assumptions similar to the kind associated with participation in Medicap policies, you find that private insurance can make a difference. It is not a total solution. It should not be one, but there is a lot of potential there, potential that will maximize choice, reward efficiencies in the system, and encourage development of a responsive system that meets the needs of the elderly.

XVIII. The Need for an Integrated System and Attention to the Uninsured

Remarks of Bruce Vladeck

Uninsured Children

At the risk of playing semantic games, we have given lip service to the issue of 11 million uninsured children, which to my way of thinking is a catastrophe. Children in this country are dying of treatable diseases because they do not have health insurance, and that is a fact. I think that is much more important than everything else we have talked about today. For most of us, worrying about that is not our job, but I hope everybody will at least feel a little embarrassed about it before we move on to talk about other things.

This is not a problem affecting Japanese children, or Taiwanese children, or German children. Uwe Reinhardt says that this very fact should disqualify us from the right to describe ourselves as citizens of a civilized nation, and I think he is right.

Even in terms of a calculus of social cost-benefit, and of preventable developmental delay that is now occurring in children throughout this country, we should not be concentrating on the elderly's health care cost at the expense of uninsured children.

Nevertheless, I think Peter Libassi is quite right: what we are talking about is not catastrophic health insurance. We are not talking about the most important issue in health care. Instead, we are talking about the issue of protecting the assets of middle-class families, as they or their families reach the age when they need long-term care.

I do think that there is a real issue of priorities here but, if we are talking about asset protection, I think it has been discussed from a strange perspective.

There is one school of thought that would argue that the problem of financing long-term care is essentially one of income adequacy for older women. These are the people who use long-term care. Long-term care clients are disproportionately widows, divorcées, or never married women in their 80s. They are people who have, until recently, perhaps not gotten their fair share as survivors under the Social Security system or under the private pension system.

We have begun to address some of those issues a little better, I think, over the last several years, but if we address them more directly, we might benefit a lot of individuals who need long-term care and provide more funds for long-term care as well as benefitting a number of people who will never need long-term care.

Similarly, the whole question of prefunding of benefits, whether it is under a payroll tax system or a private system, seems to me to get to what is really a very important issue, the national savings rate, which Harry Garber raised.

We have a real crisis in this society, in terms of international competitiveness, in the way we do a whole variety of things. I think that is not unrelated to the relative tax burden on the population, but that is a different issue. It is strange to address an issue that I think is really very central, such as the national savings rate, through the prism of substituting insurance-based rather than asset liquidation-based financing for 1.5 million people a year who enter nursing homes.

Employment-Related Benefits Less Widely Available

As a final prefatory point, I am pleased to hear about the increase in availability of private long-term care insurance through the work place because I do think that the issue of protecting assets for households is a legitimate one, and people ought to have opportunities to enter into such arrangements. However, Art Lifson and I were talking about how it would be a year and a half from now before people figure out whether the pension funds that were overfunded before the stock market dropped are still overfunded. That is assuming the market settles down by then. Everything I see having to do with employment-related benefits suggests, in fact, that they have become less widely available in recent years, rather than more widely available.

I believe that the penetration of private pension protection peaked a couple of years ago and has been on a plateau ever since, after having grown continuously since the time of Taft-Hartley Act. Maybe when some of the new COBRA and tax law changes go into effect, that will reverse, but I am skeptical, given what has happened in the labor market. Obviously, the proportion of private employees covered by health insurance has fallen in recent years.

So, I find it a little strange to say that we are going to develop this broad-scale new benefit at the same time that we are reducing all sorts of other benefits, some of which have to do with children and other age groups as well.

226

Destigmatizing Medicaid

Having said this much, let me make three more points.

First, we have catastrophic and long-term care insurance for much of the population under the Medicaid program. It is a strange kind of insurance, however, because essentially there is a 100 percent co-payment until almost all of your money is spent, then there is no copayment.*

What we are, in fact, talking about is a variety of mechanisms, such as a two-year waiting period, a national entitlement with some sort of up-front cost sharing or continuous cost sharing, that will change the nature of deductibles and coinsurance under public financing so that families are not faced with a potentially catastrophic liquidation of their children's estates. People will be able to approach some of these issues more rationally. I think there is a lot to be said for that.

But I want to go back to what I think is a more important issue for a moment, because I think there is something to be said for the uninsured, nonelderly population as well, and I would like to bring that to people's attention.

If you are concerned about those 37 million people, 20 million of whom have a connection to the work force, there is a great deal of discussion about a variety of private initiatives of one kind or another. My calculation suggests that for a family of four that is headed by an individual who works full-time at the minimum wage and lives in a state where no supplemental cash assistance is available, a typical moderately good private health insurance plan would account for 40 percent of the household's gross income. That means that this is not a question of insurance availability, or forming appropriate groups, or marketing insurance among employees. It is just not affordable for low-income markets, which implies to me that we are going to continue to need public subsidy. One approach to building public subsidy is to recognize that there is a pretty good program in place for half of the poor people in the United States; and if a way could be found to partially subsidize care from the private sector for the other half, we could probably expand coverage extensively. This is the same thing we have been talking about in terms of a part private, part public long-term care insurance program.

To make such coverage available, however, we must destigmatize Medicaid. I think that there is likely to be more discussion and some

---

*Editor's note: Under the Medicare Catastrophic Coverage Act of 1988, the income of the spouse of an institutionalized, Medicaid eligible individual would be protected up to a specified amount.

experimentation along these lines. At least in this way, perhaps, our concerns about the financing of long-term care can contribute something to the more important problem of 37 million uninsured Americans.

Medicare and Long-Term Care

We must also recognize the support of the Medicare program. Both Part A and Part B (SMI) are already expending a great deal of money on long-term care services and on other services for long-term care clients. Five percent of all Medicare beneficiaries are in a nursing home today, and those beneficiaries, in the course of a year, are going to account for 15 or 20 percent of the Part A inpatient days.

If we had more rational systems of organization and financing, it is believed—and there is some evidence to demonstrate it—that we could probably save some of those Part A monies. It is clear to anybody who has actually worked in the long-term care system that the boundary between the Medicare system and the other financing systems increases costs in many instances and causes real pain and difficulty for many beneficiaries.

It is a particularly dramatic problem these days in terms of home care. I know in New York City of hundreds of Medicare beneficiaries who are getting six hours a week of Medicare home care and 12 hours a week of other home care, from different workers, under different supervision—same client, same case—because of that kind of boundary problem. And the aggregate expenditure is greater than it needs to be.

So the administrators of the Medicare program are already involved with this problem in a variety of ways. There is a great deal to be said, at a minimum, for full integration of the Medicare program as it now exists and long-term care. If this is not done, money will be spent unnecessarily and people will not receive the kind of service they ought to have.

It is both a financial issue and a service issue, and even if we decided that we are not worried about the dollars that come out of the private sector in this regard, I think we ought to be worried about the impact on beneficiaries.

Infrastructures for long-term care are better in some communities than some observers would suggest. But I would also suggest that in those communities, as well as in others that have not gotten that far, the principal barrier to improvement is the way in which the Medicare program treats the relationship between inpatient hospital care and nursing home care as distinguished from various community-based services. If we are going to rationalize the system and develop the infrastructure, Medicare is a major player whether it is providing a "long-term care benefit" or not, and accommodations must be made to that fact.

Issues of Home Care Quality

One additional point. I do not believe that home care is as simple as some suggest. If you want to see a catastrophe, go out and see how difficult it is for some Medicare beneficiaries to receive home care, and that includes patients waiting in hospitals for arrangements to be made.

In New York City, where through Medicare, Medicaid, and private resources we provide more home care than most of the rest of the country, there are no weekend home care workers available for Medicare-certified patients who are waiting in hospitals.

The only reason we have not yet seen scandals in the home health industry that would far exceed the nursing home scandals of a decade ago is that the incidents take place behind closed doors, in people's apartments. We have a real crisis with regard to the people employed in this field, their training, the way they are paid, how they are supervised, and the quality of service the clients receive. And no one is responsible.

We do not have adequate standards or adequate enforcement, and we have an absolute catastrophe out there. I am concerned that, given the current state of the home care system in many communities, when private insurers start paying for this benefit, in addition to helping to make the situation worse, they are going to create all kinds of liabilities for themselves. I would just warn you about this before the discussion continues much further.

Lastly, I would point out that if you have to spend a certain amount for a service, whether the service is nursing home care, community-based care, or whatever, from an analytic point of view, it should not matter whether this money is called tax dollars or private dollars. But, in fact, what 90 percent of the discussion is really about these days is the wish of those responsible for raising and spending tax dollars to appear as if they are not spending public funds.

Data from other countries and from various experiences in the health care system in the United States suggest that in some instances, if the money were not necessarily all public or all private, but were all funneled through a single agency in a given community, the total amount needed would be substantially less than if the money continued to come from many different places.

A Fragmented, Piecemeal, and Inadequate System?

And yet it seems to me that, for ideological reasons, we are going to make worse a system that is already excessively fragmented, piece-meal, and inadequate. That has major financial implications, and also major adverse implications for the quality of care that people are getting.

Although most of the money is there already, our nation has an affordability problem in terms of long-term care. It is irresponsible to seek to provide people with more and better long-term care without trying to provide it at the least possible cost, and this cannot be accomplished by encouraging further fragmentation of the market on the buyer side.

The least possible cost is to have as monopolistic a purchaser as you can on the buyer side—government or private. Someone has to do it or otherwise, as has been the experience with hospitals and physicians, the cost of providers' services will become prohibitive.

This is not an analytic issue; it is a political and ideological issue.

XIX. Public versus Private Insurance

REMARKS OF EDWARD F. HOWARD

Measuring a Catastrophic Expense by Its Impact on People

The notion of catastrophic expense, as has been emphasized in several of the papers, has to be measured in terms of the impact on the people for whom it is a catastrophe. I am told day after day, that for Mrs. Rockefeller, the cost of care for Alzheimer's disease is not a catastrophe. Health care expense is catastrophic when it is a financial catastrophe.

About 26 percent of elderly persons with incomes of $10,000 or less have expenditures on health care of greater than 15 percent of this income, which is a common amount used to measure a threshold for catastrophic expense.

What I am trying to emphasize is that there is, in both the private and public sector solutions sometimes offered, a lack of focus on the people who are suffering the catastrophic impact that we allegedly are trying to handle.

With respect to Steven Grossman's observation about long-term care not necessarily being catastrophic in expense, let me offer two observations. One has to do with a study that came out of New York recently in preparation for a debate on spousal impoverishment legislation at the state level. The conclusion reached was that it was not going to be very costly for the state to provide asset protection for the spouses of nursing home residents, because those nursing home residents were coming from hospitals and they had spent all their assets anyway. There wasn't anything to protect, so they could be allowed to keep all they had at very little cost.

The other observation has to do with costs that do not show up in home care bills: the cost of the spouse who has to retire; the cost of the health care of that spouse when her health declines as a result of the burdens; and the cost to the families, who have their lives disrupted, their careers disrupted, their children's education disrupted.

A Public-Private Mix in Long-Term Care Services

And, finally, going way out on a limb, I predict that there will be a public-private mix in long-term care services in the future. I hope the public side will predominate.

There is a question of trust raised in those poll results about private sector versus public sector administration of this program, a concern that private insurance companies might compromise quality to save on costs.

There is also the question that Phyllis Borzi raised about the nature of entitlement, whether it is public or private, and whether there will be a broad basic benefit package. There will be standards, whether they are government-administered or government-set, and there will be a public role in setting those standards, I believe. With respect to private insurance, it is clear that we are going to have a long shake-down period, no matter how many inducements are placed in the tax code or in public policy.

Private Insurance as an Experimental Offering

As Mr. McCormack said in an earlier chapter, private insurance is an experimental offering. We are talking about many factors: the adverse selection, denial, the lack of proportionality, and the very long period between the time a person starts paying for these benefits and the time he or she receives them in any significant respect. We are not talking particularly about poor people. They are protected, although imperfectly, by the Medicaid program, although not very many get coverage in some states.

In Texas, for example, if you have income of $650 a month, no matter how badly you need nursing home care or how much you "spend down," you do not qualify for Medicaid. And the very rich, obviously, have no need for private insurance.

Low- and moderate-income elders have the greatest stake in this debate and, obviously, private insurance is going to develop outside of that low and moderate need. The extent to which it dips down to cover a great percentage of the population represents a tradeoff that, frankly, I have some reservations about, because of the drain on resources and the question of political will. If a substantially private market is reaching people who can pay the taxes and vote for people who can enact programs, the chance for a public sector program that meets low income and moderate income needs is reduced.

The resistance of employers and employees to making this a bargaining issue, along with the other factors that we talked about, brings to mind the well-worn axiom: "everybody's business is nobody's business." That is where I think the debate on long-term care is taking us.

XX. Part Five Discussion

The Value of Home Care

Ms. BORZI: Steve Grossman's comment that long-term care issues are different from acute care is certainly correct, and I agree that long-term care is not inherently catastrophic. But I am quite concerned about his rationale for placing virtually no value on home health care.

Several times he said it does not cost anything or the cost is very little. He articulated the premise over and over. To the extent that people tend to put little or no value on the kind of health care delivery system that is provided by families, that contributes to the problem, and it is not part of the solution.

In trying to deal with the question of long-term care or health care generally, if we continue to put little or no value on the kind of services that the family provides, then there will be little or no incentive for the family to continue to provide those services. It certainly is not correct to say that because we do not have a home health care worker coming to this family, it is therefore a low or no-cost option.

I do not think anyone who has been in a caregiving situation would ever describe the home health care option as one that involves little or no cost. I do not remember the exact percentage from the Travelers' survey, but there were at least some respondents who said that they put in at least 80 hours a week in a caregiving role, in addition to their full-time job.

QUESTION FROM THE AUDIENCE: What is the cost of that?

MR. GROSSMAN: There is a contradiction. On the one hand, I have said that we ought to look at the dollars involved, the catastrophic expenses. The dollar trail does not lead, except for a very small number of people, to home care. But I think I also said that if we design a long-term care system in which we turn the low or no cost services that families provide into dollars, we are going to have an even more difficult time funding that system.

So, if that was not interpreted as support for home care and a realization that it involves enormous sacrifice, I would apologize because I certainly do agree that home care is important and should be reinforced.

235

Who Pays the Cost of Home Care?

MS. BORZI: You are right. That is a contradiction in terms because I see the total cost being the same. The question is, who pays it? And you are saying that you are willing to continue a system in which the same type of share, a larger share, is being borne by the family because that does not show up in real dollars. It is real dollars because, for every dollar that the family provides, it is less that someone else has to provide, but that does not mean the costs go away.

MR. VLADECK: I hope you do not want to let yourself be accused of a perverse extension of the argument that was made before—that the federal government thinks of all dollars as belonging to it unless it lets you keep them.

MS. BORZI: No, I did not say the federal government.

MR. GROSSMAN: I do not think we want to assume that all care that is provided translates into dollars, and people have to be rewarded. People provide care basically out of compassion and caring and because they are doing what they feel is right in their relationship with the individual needing assistance. We want to support that, but care should be taken not to wind up paying for all those services that people are now providing free because that would further exacerbate the in-the-system dollar problem.

MS. BORZI: I am not disagreeing with that. I am simply saying that one needs to recognize that every expenditure does not show up in terms of a cash outlay.

MR. GROSSMAN: I quite agree. But its worth being clear here: actively encouraging home care and family responsibility are a valid theme not entirely reconcilable with dealing with the financial cost of nursing home care.

MR. VLADECK: I want to make a narrower point in this regard. The issue of the economic cost of the family contribution is important and very complicated, but it is not the point I want to make. The point I do want to make is, if you are the federal government and even if, for hypothetical purposes, you are obligated by law to provide a benefit and you do not provide it, it does not cost you anything.

Now, one of the reasons we have spent so little money on home care is because people do not get it, even when they need it. So, I think it is important not to be misled by that "technical data" problem.

236

A Family Stress Problem

MR. ROTHER: It is misleading to look at this whole thing in terms of catastrophic. I really think that is the wrong framework to start with. In the poll AARP-Villers conducted, we found that real people in the real world do not view this problem primarily as a financial one.

They view it primarily as a family stress problem, and the financial part is secondary—still important, but secondary.

The prediction is that we are going to see every single declared presidential candidate proposing some kind of policy for long-term care. And I certainly hope that, in addition, they will have something to say about the uninsured as well.

Sorting through Priorities

MR. LANE: I just wanted to commend Bruce Vladeck for helping us sort through some priorities. As a nation, we do have a long list of things that need to be done and a very small checking account to devote to them.

Recently I read an article on age and dependency that discussed how we have separated children from the aged in terms of social welfare, and how there is an increasing dichotomy in policy decisions. As a person who had been advocate in the aging field for a long time, it is very difficult for me to say that it may not be our turn. I find few flaws in Robert Friedland's broad vision and a strong sense of moral commitment towards it. However, as a pragamatist I lean toward Peter Libassi in saying that it may not be our turn. Some positive decisions are being made that are beginning to focus attention on issues of asset-targeted and untargeted protections when it comes to insurance or other savings devices. I believe that the concept of a health security platform may have begun and ended after two decades of discussion, and that we missed the chance to reform Medicaid when it was a viable, realistic option because the debate became politically polarized. I caution against further polarization of this issue and against moving on to other concerns and postponing action on long-term care until the 1990s, in the hope that by then we will have a better idea of what the market is for insurance.

The Relationship of Home Care to Nursing Homes

MS. YOUNG: Mr. Grossman, did you factor in the number of elderly persons who may be going into nursing homes, which are much more expensive than home care because, with families working, there is no caregiver at home. There is no one to hire or the means to pay for a home health worker to come in for several hours a day to look after a grandparent. So the elderly, incontinent person winds up in a nursing home at a much greater cost.

MR. GROSSMAN: Let me try to address that in two ways. In a scientific sense, there is much we can do. For example, think of the advances that are sure to be made to help the problem of incontinence and I have high hopes for advances against Alzheimer's disease. Ten or fifteen years from now, there will likely be a different and maybe smaller problem.

In terms of the relationship of home care to nursing homes, I can tell you what I believe and I can tell you what the studies would probably show. What I believe is that there are some real savings there. I do not know what the offset cost is of a broad-based program that would pay for home care, when you would be paying for many activities that would take place anyway, regardless of the incentive.

I need to point out that virtually all the studies the Department of Health and Human Services has done fail to show any significant savings for home care in terms of its ability to displace nursing home care. Families more often send individuals to nursing homes when they can no longer bear the physical and emotional burdens of home care than they do for financial reasons.

MS. YOUNG: But can they get help? That is the question that no one seems to ask.

MR. GROSSMAN: There is help available for the frail elderly who live alone, with family far away, although more needs to be available.

One of the interesting factors that we picked up in the AARP-Villers study is that about 50 percent of the elderly live a considerable distance from their children. The prevailing assumption everyone makes is that the children have moved away from the parents. In fact, many parents have moved away from their children and live in Florida and the Southwest. Those states are going to have significant problems. To some extent they already do and they will have more as people who moved there in their 50s or 60s grow older.

MR. SALISBURY: Ms. Young, I interpreted Bruce Vladeck's comments vis-à-vis the problem in New York City of finding enough qualified people to be evidence that the issue you are raising has been identified and exists. But the structure is not necessarily there to deal with it. I read into his comment that even if more people could stay in their homes, there are tremendous liability, regulation, and control issues that affect the quality of the care they would receive there versus the care in a nursing home.

Ms. YOUNG: Has anyone done a study on whether or not the shortage of home-health care workers is propelling more people into nursing homes, and whether that solution is actually more expensive than training and paying home care workers?

MR. GROSSMAN: I agree with Bruce Vladeck that there is much more we can do in home care that is worth doing. Somehow I have been interpreted as being very negative on home care, and I would stress that in my view we should not turn our back on it by any means. There are things to be done.

MR. VLADECK: I imagine you could always say that the people who cannot get home care either stay in the hospital, if the hospital is responsible, long past the time they should, or go home without care, if the hospital is not responsible.

Taking Care of the Young as Well as the Old

Just one other word on Laurence Lane's comments, because I was afraid we would fall into this trap. I think the first priority has to be providing care for children who are not getting enough. But I think this is a rich society, and I very much reject the notion that we somehow have to trade off the needs of the elderly for those of young people. I would summarize my feelings about that by saying that my estimate is that the average annual inflation in health care costs, at current levels, holding service volume constant, is between $35 billion and $40 billion. That is one year's growth increment, with no net increase in service. One might say this is revenue to providers. And you could pay all the long-term care and all the comprehensive child health, and still have some money left over out of that amount. This is the issue on which we should be focusing, not trading off one group's need against another's.

MR. FLEMING: When I was leaving the house this morning, I explained to my wife what the agenda would be, and she said to me, "What's your solution?" I said, "I don't have a solution," and as I was going out the door, she said, "Well, maybe you'll find one."

I do not think we have found a solution, but I think bringing all of us together is essential. After spending a lifetime in employee benefits, I would just once like to be out in front of a problem, recognize the problem, and begin to find the solution before a catastrophe occurs. When that happens, catastrophic solutions are given, and seldom are they worthwhile.

Appendix A
Forum Participants

Moderator
Dallas L. Salisbury
President
Employee Benefit Research
    Institute

Speakers and Authors
Robert M. Ball
Consultant on Social Security,
    Health and Welfare Policy

Charles Betley
Research Assistant
Employee Benefit Research
    Institute

Deborah J. Chollet
Senior Research Associate
Employee Benefit Research
    Institute

Robert B. Friedland
Research Associate
Employee Benefit Research
    Institute

Mary Jo Gibson
Health Policy Analyst
    Public Policy Institute
American Association of Retired
    Persons

Steven A. Grossman
Deputy Assistant Secretary for
    Health (Planning and
    Evaluation)
U.S. Department of Health and
    Human Services

Edward F. Howard
Public Policy Coordinator
The Villers Foundation

Karen Ignagni
Assistant Director
Department of Occupational
    Safety, Health and Social
    Security
AFL-CIO

Laurence F. Lane
Vice President for Regulatory
    Affairs
InSpeech, Inc.

F. Peter Libassi
Senior Vice President, Corporate
    Communications
The Travelers Companies

Stephen R. McConnell
Coordinator
Long Term Care '88

John J. McCormack
Executive Vice President
Teachers Insurance and Annuity
    Association/College Retirement
    Equities Fund

Janet A. Myder
Director of Special Programs
American Health Care Association

Thomas O'Brien
Dean, School of Management
University of Massachusetts

John C. Rother
Director of Legislation, Research
    and Public Policy
American Association of Retired
    Persons

Theresa Varner
Health Policy Analyst
    Public Policy Institute
American Association of Retired
    Persons

Bruce C. Vladeck
President
United Hospital Fund

Richard Woodbury
Graduate Student
Harvard University

Leon Wyszewianski
School of Public Health
University of Michigan

Participants

B. K. Atrostic
Financial Economist
Office of Tax Analysis
U.S. Department of the Treasury

Mark C. Blackwell
Director of Employee Benefits
BATUS Inc.

Phyllis Borzi
Counsel for Pensions
Subcommittee on Labor-
  Management Relations
House Education and Labor
  Committee

Steven Brostoff
Washington Editor
National Underwriter

Kenneth E. Brunke, Jr.
Executive Director
Callan Investments Institute

William S. Cartwright
Chief, Demography & Economics
  Office
National Institute of Aging

Isabelle Claxton
Business & Health

Barbara Coleman
American Association of Retired
  Persons

Ray S. Crabtree
Senior Vice President
The Principal Financial Group

Carol Cronin
Vice President, Policy
Washington Business Group on
  Health

Richard E. Curtis
Director of Health Policy Studies
National Governors Association

Ginny Felice
Executive Director, Special
  Commission on Elderly Health
  Care
Commonwealth of Massachusetts

Rhona Fischer
Research Associate
Intergovernmental Health Policy
  Project
George Washington University

John Fleming
Administrative Director
Bakery and Confectionery Union
  and Industry International
  Health Benefits and Pension
  Funds

Beth Fuchs
Analyst in Social Legislation
Congressional Research Service

Margaret M. Gagliardi
Vice President, Compensation and
  Benefits
American Express, Travel Related
  Services Company, Inc.

Harry Garber
Vice Chairman
The Equitable Life Assurance
  Society of the United States

Marcy Lynn Gross
Policy Analyst
U.S. Department of Health and
  Human Services

Edmund Haislmaier
Policy Analyst
The Heritage Foundation

Donald P. Harrington
Corporate Vice President
AT&T

Robert C. Hendrickson
Corporate Director, Employee
  Benefits
The Sherwin-Williams Company

Lorraine K. Hiatt
Research Associate
National Health Council, Inc.

Robert F. Hickox
Co-Publisher
Enterprise Communications

Justina F. Holmes
Coordinator, Health Care
E. I. du Pont de Nemours &
    Company, Inc.

Joseph Holtzer
Managing Director
William M. Mercer-Meidinger-
    Hansen, Incorporated

Michael Hoon
Legislative Assistant
Senator Malcolm Wallop

Neil J. Horgan
Director, Compensation and
    Benefits
Sun Company, Inc.

Paul H. Jackson
Vice President and Director
The Wyatt Company

Jeanne F. Kardos
Director, Employee Benefits
Southern New England
    Telecommunications

John K. Kittredge
Executive Vice President
The Prudential Insurance
    Company of America

Robert F. Leonard, Jr.
District Staff Manager, Benefits
    Planning
NYNEX Corporation

Marion Ein Lewin
Senior Staff Officer
Institute of Medicine
National Academy of Sciences

Arthur Lifson
Vice President
Equicor, Inc.

Dave Lindeman
Principal Analyst
Congressional Budget Office

Rob Lively
Legislative Representative
National Rural Electric
    Cooperative Association

Michael J. Mahoney, F.S.A.
Milliman & Robertson, Inc.

Richard G. Merrill
Executive Vice President
The Prudential Insurance
    Company of America

Warren L. Moser
Vice President, Strategic Planning
    & Product Containment
    Development
United Health Care, Inc.

Maureen D. Mullen
Director, Employee Benefits
    Division
Aetna Life & Casualty

Richard Murphy
Director of Research
Buck Consultants, Inc.

Gino Nalli
Consultant
The Wyatt Company

Diane D. O'Brien
Executive Director, Human
    Resources Policy and Planning
Pacific Telesis Group

Robert Patterson
Senior Vice President, Finance
    and Legal
Pennsylvania Blue Shield

Robert D. Paul
Vice Chairman
Martin E. Segal Company

Stephen Press
Vice President for Acquisitions
Meditrust

Charlene C. Quinn
Director, Office of Policy Planning
and Liaison
U.S. Department of Health and
Human Services

Michael J. Reardon
Second Vice President, Issue
Management
UNUM Life Insurance Company

Michael J. Reynolds
President
Frank B. Hall Consulting
Company

Carole Thompson Roberts
Director, Federal Government
Affairs
The Travelers Companies

Michael F. Rodgers
Deputy Executive Vice President
American Association of Homes
for the Aging

Melvyn J. Rodrigues
Manager, Benefit Plans Research
and Compliance
Atlantic Richfield Company

Michael J. Romig
Associate General Counsel
American Council of Life
Insurance

Gail P. Schaeffer
General Director, Long-Term Care
John Hancock Financial Services

Jerry Schiff
Financial Economist
Office of Tax Analysis
U.S. Department of the Treasury

Burt Schorr
Editor
Health Policy Week

Charles L. Schulze
Director, Personnel
Cincinnati Bell Telephone
Company

Nancy Simmons
Editor, *Benefits Today*

Jesse M. Smith, Jr.
Associate Executive Director
American Compensation
Association

Stephen A. Somers
Senior Program Officer
Robert Wood Johnson Foundation

Denise Spence
Senior Research Analyst
Brookings Institution

Amy Stevens
Vice President, Pension and
Insurance Department
Goldman, Sachs & Co.

R. N. Swilley
Director, Benefits
BellSouth Corporation

Lawrence H. Thompson
Chief Economist
U.S. General Accounting Office

Thomas Ucko
Vice President, National Benefits
Consulting Division
Corroon & Black Corporation

Roger L. Vaughn
Executive Vice President
Booke & Company

David M. Walker
Assistant Secretary, Pension and
Welfare Benefits Administration
U.S. Department of Labor

Leah Young
Journalist
Journal of Commerce

244

245

Appendix B
Report to Congress and the Secretary by the Task Force on Long-Term Health Care Policies*

The challenge of meeting the needs of our disabled and aging population requires immediate attention. Few individuals can finance an extended nursing home stay or other long-term care services entirely out of their assets and incomes. Many people, however, may be able to provide for nursing home and other long-term care services through buying long-term insurance.

At age 65 people are estimated to have more than a 43 percent risk of entering a nursing home some time during the rest of their lives. However, financing long-term care is not just a problem for older persons. In the year 2000, 40 percent of functionally dependent Americans will be less than 65 years old. Besides the high cost of financing institutional care, disabled and older persons living in the community will need long-term care services to remain at home.

The Task Force on Long-Term Health Care Policies [hereafter Task Force] strongly recommends that both public and private sectors take steps immediately to encourage expansion of private financing for long-term care services through long-term care insurance. Even during the Task Force's deliberations, and partly in response to its initiatives, the development of long-term care insurance has moved forward, but the pace of development needs to accelerate. The Task Force offers its recommendations as a blueprint for more rapidly developing and expanding a private system for financing long-term care.

Long-term care includes a wide range of medical and support services for people who suffer physical or mental disorders causing functional limitation or disability and therefore need assistance for an extended period to maintain or promote functional well-being. Long-term care ranges from informal in-home services to institutional skilled nursing.

---

*Editor's note: This is the executive summary of the *Report to Congress and the Secretary by the Task Force on Long-Term Health Care Policies* prepared in accordance with Section 9601 of the Consolidated Omnibus Budget Reconciliation Act of 1985, U.S. Department of Health and Human Services, Health Care Financing Administration, Washington, DC: Government Printing Office, 1987.

Spending on long-term care has grown rapidly and will continue to grow as the population ages. Almost half the institutional costs for long-term care are paid directly out-of-pocket, while less than 2 percent is paid through insurance.

The statute creating the Task Force requested recommendations for action in the areas of education, market development, and consumer protection to improve and foster the growth of long-term care insurance.

The Task Force accepted the definition of long-term care insurance adopted by the National Association of Insurance Commissioners (NAIC) in their Long-Term Care Insurance Model Act (Model Act). This definition requires insurance to offer benefits for not less than 12 consecutive months in a setting other than an acute care unit·of a hospital. The Task Force added explanatory notes to the definition to clarify certain points: 1) services are covered in various settings—at home or in the community, as well as in institutions; 2) long-term care insurance does not duplicate Medicare coverage for those eligible; 3) covered services include personal care to maintain activities of daily living; 4) future policies may bring arrangements not yet envisioned; and 5) the Task Force encourages development of both the products covered by the definition and other forms of risk pooling.

Private long-term care insurance can protect people against large out-of-pocket expenses. It gives individuals the opportunity to retain choices and develop a flexible, planned response to a potentially ruinous event that will confront many people over 65 as well as many disabled people under 65. Insurance offers the most cost effective, collective approach to meeting financial risks that often devastate individuals.

The Task Force believes a broad market for long-term care insurance can and should be developed. While very few disabled and older persons have obtained long-term care insurance, no other private financing mechanism appears to offer a more effective and viable means of meeting long-term care costs.

The Task Force acknowledges that private long-term care insurance cannot provide a total solution for financing long-term care. For the foreseeable future long-term care will continue to be provided by formal and informal caregivers, in institutional, home, and community settings, and financed by a mixture of public and private expenditures. When the task force reviewed integrated public/private approaches, especially those significantly expanding government financial support for catastrophic episodes of long-term care, it concluded that more information was needed to determine the viability of a joint public/private approach.

The Task Force identified and analyzed market factors that promise to stimulate an active private long-term care insurance market with attractive and affordable products and, at the same time, provide reasonable protection for consumers. In the judgment of the task force, the critical factors are these:

- Public Awareness—Consumers need to be more aware of several key topics: 1) the absence of long-term care coverage under Medicare, Medicare supplement insurance, and most acute care insurance and prepaid health programs; 2) the potential costs of long-term care over their lifetime; 3) the range, cost, and availability of long-term care insurance products; and 4) the advantages and limitations of various insurance features. In particular, the Federal government has a responsibility to inform Social Security beneficiaries that Medicare does not cover long-term care services.

- Consumer Protection—The Task Force found that the Long-Term Insurance Model Act developed by the National Association of Insurance Commissioners provides a sound basis for balancing the interests of product development with adequate protection for consumers. However, greater consumer protection can be provided through more stringent requirements for renewability of individual long-term care insurance policies and through the regulation of the reserves for continuing care retirement communities.

- Market Development—The absence of basic data on the use of long-term care insurance by an insured population and the need to define benefit levels present problems for insurance companies in designing products that meet certain needs: 1) cover services in expanded settings like homes and communities; 2) prevent overuse of services (induced demand); and 3) avoid creating a risk pool weighted too heavily to those most likely to require long-term care (adverse selection). The Task Force generally concluded that insurance companies must be given latitude to experiment with benefit design and utilization controls if they are to develop products that will be affordable and attractive to consumers.

- Expansion of the Market through Employer-Sponsored Long-term Care Insurance—Offering long-term care insurance through employment has the greatest potential to cover large numbers of people, but penetrating this market will require overcoming impediments and providing incentives.

- Tax Incentives—Existing rules must be clarified in several respects: the tax treatment of reserves for long-term care insurance and interest on those reserves and the tax treatment of long-term care insurance in general. Tax incentives are especially important to encourage development of long-term care insurance through employment-based plans and vested retirement funds. Compared to other approaches, employment-based plans would make more attractive and affordable products available and extend coverage to the largest number of people.

Efforts of the NAIC have significantly advanced the work of the Task Force in developing recommendations to assure responsible marketing practices and prevent sales abuses. In adopting the Model Act, the NAIC has established an appropriate vehicle for protecting consumers. The Task Force was able to further NAIC efforts by developing an additional recommendation to give Insurance Commissioners greater authority over cancellation and renewability of long-term care insurance policies.

The Congress charged the Task Force to recommend ways to assure a reasonable relationship between premiums and benefits, and this task presented marked difficulties. The NAIC draft regulations dated June 22, 1987, rely on loss ratio to test premium reasonableness, but the Task Force concluded that this test is of limited use at present. Further developing actuarial tables on frequency and duration of nursing home stay and utilization may prove to be more helpful in judging the real value of long-term care insurance.

The Task Force adopted 41 recommendations. Taken together, they provide practical directions for strengthening long-term care financing through private insurance. They vary in difficulty of implementation, effect on the issues, cost effectiveness, political acceptability, and budget impact. Particularly important recommendations cover seven areas, and their implementation should command the highest priority.

1. Inform consumers that Medicare, Medigap, and acute health care insurance do not cover long-term care. The Department of Health and Human Services should communicate directly to all current and new Social Security beneficiaries the exact nature and limitations of Medicare long-term care coverage, as well as available alternatives. Effective communication will require developing appropriate information and referral capabilities.

2. Encourage states to adopt the National Association of Insurance Commissioners' Long-Term Care Insurance Model Act. A number of states have already adopted the Model Act, and all other states are strongly encouraged to do the same. The task force believes, however, that the cancellation provision should be more limited than permitted in the Model Act.

3. Promote the availability of long-term care insurance through employment. Offering long-term care insurance through employment is an effective way to make attractive, affordable coverage available to large groups of working-age people. A number of approaches promise to help

accomplish this objective. Tax incentives and encouragement of employer cooperation will be essential to these efforts. At a minimum, the present restrictions on buying long-term care insurance through cafeteria plans and flexible spending accounts should be removed.

4. Develop long-term care insurance financing through vested pension funds. Both before and after retirement, individuals should be permitted to use vested pension and retirement savings (including IRAs, Keogh plans, and others) to purchase long-term care insurance. Transfers from such funds should not be taxed or subject to penalties.

5. Use Federal and state tax codes to encourage the purchase of long-term care insurance. Most desirable would be broad-based measures that effectively encourage purchase of long-term care insurance without unduly reducing government revenues. The most important incentive in lowering the cost of long-term care insurance depends on clarifying whether tax exempt status applies to long-term care insurance reserves held by insurers and to the investment earnings credited to them.

6. Encourage new approaches to determine eligibility for long-term care insurance benefits. The level-of-care and service definitions currently in use are unreliable in determining eligibility for long-term care insurance benefits. The Task Force believes that developing need assessment systems, based on ability to perform activities of daily living, offers a useful alternative in deciding eligibility for benefits.

7 Encourage greater cooperation in the collection and sharing of long-term care data.

The Task Force, with the cooperation of the Department of Health and Human Services and the Veterans Administration, has taken steps to increase the sharing of Federal data and recommends further Federal, State, and private efforts to improve the quality and availability of actuarial data.

Appendix C
The Medicare Catastrophic Coverage Act
of 1988

The following pages relate the final provisions agreed to by the Conference Committee of the U.S. Congress on H.R. 2470, The Medicare Catastrophic Coverage Act of 1988, as explained in the May 31, 1988 summary of the Conference Agreement.

Provisions Relating to Part A

1. Inpatient Hospital Services

   a. *Inpatient Hospital Deductible*—The inpatient hospital deductible would apply only to a beneficiary's first period of continuous hospitalization beginning in a calendar year.

   However, if a beneficiary paid a deductible during December of a calendar year, the beneficiary would not be required to pay an additional deductible for a hospitalization beginning in January of the following year. The deductible is estimated to be approximately $564 in 1989.

   b. *Elimination of Day Limitation on Inpatient Hospital Services*—The Medicare limits on payment for days of inpatient hospital care (90 days of inpatient hospital care plus a lifetime reserve of 60 days) would be eliminated so that Medicare would pay for an unlimited number of hospital days for covered services. The 190-day lifetime limit on inpatient psychiatric hospital services would be retained.

   c. *Elimination of Coinsurance Amounts for Inpatient Hospital Services*—The current hospital inpatient coinsurance amounts for days 61 through 90 and coinsurance for the 60 lifetime reserve days would be eliminated.

   d. *Elimination of "Spell of Illness"*—The "spell of illness" methodology would be eliminated for determining: the number of hospital days Medicare would cover, the skilled nursing facility coinsurance and the Part A blood deductible.

   e. *Adjustments in Payments for Inpatient Hospital Services*—When adjusting the Medicare hospital payment system, the Secretary of Health and Human Services (HHS) would be required to take into account the reductions in beneficiary payments to hospitals because of the elimination of the day limitation.

   The Secretary, when appropriate, would adjust the payment rates under the prospective payment system (PPS), (including the outlier cutoff points, and the weighting factors), and would be required on a hospital-specific basis to adjust the target amounts for paying non-PPS hospitals.

  f. *Chronic Ventilator-Dependent Unit Demonstration Program*—The Secretary would be required to initiate up to five projects to demonstrate the feasibility of including chronic ventilator-dependent unit services as rehabilitation services under the Medicare program. The services would be reimbursed on a cost basis as are other rehabilitation services.

2. Extended Care Services (Skilled Nursing Facility)

  a. *Coinsurance on First Eight Days*—Beneficiaries would be required to pay coinsurance amounts for the first eight days of such services in a calendar year.

  b. *Coinsurance Equal to 20 Percent*—The coinsurance amount per day would be equal to 20 percent of the national average per diem Medicare reasonable cost for a skilled nursing facility (SNF) services. The coinsurance amount is estimated to be approximately $20.50 per day in 1989.

  c. *Cover 150 Days of Care*—The Medicare program would cover 150 days of skilled nursing care services in a calendar year.

  d. *Prior Hospitalization Requirement*—The three-day prior hospitalization requirement for skilled nursing facility benefits would be eliminated effective for skilled nursing facility stays beginning on or after January 1, 1989.

3. Hospice Care

  a. *Extending Day Limit*—The Medicare program would extend the hospice benefit, and reimburse a hospice, beyond the current 210-day benefit period if the beneficiary's physician or hospice director recertified that the beneficiary was still terminally ill. The current-law cap on hospice reimbursement would be maintained.

4. Blood Deductible

  a. *Change Blood-Deductible Requirement*—A Medicare beneficiary would be responsible for payment of a deductible equal to the expenses incurred for the first three pints of whole blood (or equivalent quantities of packed red blood cells) furnished each calendar year. The blood deductible could be met by replacing the blood, in accordance with regulations. The Part A blood deductible would be reduced to the extent that a blood deductible had been paid under Part B.

5. Part A Premium

  a. *Recalculation*—Requires the Secretary (beginning in 1989) to establish a new Part A monthly premium amount equal to the estimated actuarial value of the Part A benefit. The premium is estimated to be $158 a month in 1989.

6. Effective Date

a. *Effective Date*—The above Part A benefits would be effective for services provided on or after January 1, 1989.

Provisions Relating to Part B

1. Limitation on Medicare Out-of-Pocket Expenses under Part B

a. *Limit Out-of-Pocket Expenses*—After a Medicare beneficiary had incurred out-of-pocket Part B covered expenses in a calendar year which exceeded the Part B catastrophic limit, (a) Medicare would be required to pay 100 percent of reasonable costs or reasonable charges for any additional Part B covered services in the year, and (b) no further deductibles would be required.

Out-of-pocket Part B expenses would be defined to include the Part B $75 deductible, the Part B blood deductible, and the 20-percent coinsurance required to be paid by beneficiaries for Part B benefits.

The Part B catastrophic limit is estimated, according to preliminary estimates by the Congressional Budget Office, to be $1,370 in 1990. The limit would be indexed so that a constant share of Medicare beneficiaries, 7.0% according to preliminary estimates by the Congressional Budget Office, would be eligible for benefits from the catastrophic limit each year.

For prepaid health care organizations paid on the basis of aggregate reasonable cost, the Secretary would be required to provide for an appropriate adjustment to their payment amounts to reflect the increase in protection as if payment were made on an individual-by-individual basis.

Medicare carriers would be required to provide individuals, who have incurred sufficient out-of-pocket expenses, to qualify for catastrophic benefits, with a notice to that effect.

b. *Institutional-Provider Limitation*—Institutional providers with agreements with the Medicare program would be prohibited from charging Medicare beneficiaries for services for which catastrophic benefit payments are made to the provider.

2. Home Health Services:

a. *Extension of Home Health Services*—The "intermittent" skilled nursing care definition for home health services would be expanded so that "daily" would be defined as up to seven days a week for up to 38 days in any given period, instead of five days a week for up to two or three weeks. Current guidelines allowing for continuation of services under unusual circumstances would be recognized.

3. Mammography Screening:

   a. *Coverage of Mammography Screening*—Mammography screening would be covered for elderly and disabled Medicare beneficiaries. For women 65 years of age and over, exams would be available every other year.

   For disabled women under 65 years of age, a baseline screening would be available between age 35 and 40; between age 40 and 49 exams would be available every other year, except high risk individuals could receive a screening each year; and between age 50 and 64 an annual screening would be available.

   The reasonable charge would be limited to the lower of $50 in 1990 indexed to the Medicare Economic Index (MEI), or the current-law fee schedule. Quality standards would be required beginning in 1990.

   By May 1, 1990, the Physician's Payment Review Commission would be directed to study and report to Congress on the appropriate payment limit and how the limit would affect access to the benefit. By the same date, the General Accounting Office (GAO) would be required to study and report on the quality of care provided by clinics providing mammography screenings.

4. Respite-Care Benefit

   a. *Coverage of In-Home Care For Certain Chronically Dependent Individuals*—In-home care for a chronically dependent individual would be provided for up to 80 hours a year. The individual would be eligible to receive such services for 12 months after the individual first meets the Part B catastrophic limit or the prescription drug deductible. A "chronically dependent individual" would be defined as someone who is dependent on a voluntary care-giver for assistance with at least two activities of daily living (eating, bathing, dressing, toileting or transferring in and out of bed or in and out of a chair).

5. Provisions Relating to Home IV-Drug Therapy

   a. *General*—Effective January 1, 1990, Medicare would cover home intravenous (IV) drugs and associated items and services (including supplies, equipment and nursing and pharmacy services).

   b. *Coverage*—All IV antibiotics would be covered initially. Other IV drugs would be covered only if the Secretary first makes a finding that such drugs generally can be safely and effectively administered in a home setting.

   c. *Deductible and Coinsurance*—There would be no deductible or coinsurance for the home IV-drug services. Covered home IV drugs, however, would be subject to the standard drug benefit deductible and to 20-percent coinsurance. The drug benefit deductible would be waived if the course of home therapy is part of a continuous course of therapy initiated in a hospital.

   d. *Payment*—Payment for home IV drugs would follow the reimbursement principles outlined in the preceding section. Payment for associated items and services would be based on a per diem fee schedule established by the Secretary. There would be limitations on referrals to a home IV provider by a physician who receives compensation from, or has an ownership interest in, the provider.

e. *Quality Assurance*—A plan of care must be developed by the physician prescribing the home IV-drug therapy. In addition, through 1993, prior approval by a PRO would be required as a condition of payment. PROs would be required to complete review determinations within one working day of the request. Home IV-drug therapy providers must meet a number of requirements to assure quality.

f. *Intermediate Sanctions*—Intermediate sanctions would be established for providers which fail to comply with certain requirements.

6. Effective Dates:

a. *Effective Date*—The above Part B benefits would be effective for services furnished on or after January 1, 1990.

Provisions Relating to Outpatient Prescription Drugs

1. Coverage and Phase-in

a. *General*—Effective January 1, 1990, Medicare would cover home intravenous (IV) therapy drugs and immunosuppressive drugs used after the first year after transplantation. Twenty-percent coinsurance would apply to IV drugs, and 50-percent coinsurance for immunosuppressives. Effective January 1, 1991, Medicare would cover all other prescription drugs subject to 50-percent coinsurance in 1991, 40-percent in 1992, and 20-percent thereafter.

b. *Coverage*—Subject to the phase-in described above, all prescription drugs marketed prior to 1938, and all prescription drugs approved by the FDA as safe and effective, would be covered.

c. *Prohibition of Formulary*—The Secretary would be prohibited from implementing a formulary to exclude from coverage any drug otherwise covered.

2. Deductible:

a. *General*—The deductible would be $550 for 1990; $600 for 1991; $652 for 1992. After 1992, the deductible would be indexed so that approximately 16.8 percent of Medicare beneficiaries would exceed the deductible limit.

b. *Special Rule for Home IV-Drug Therapy*—The deductible would be waived in the case of home IV-drug therapy initiated during a hospital admission.

3. Payment for Single-Source Drugs and Multiple-Source Drugs with a Restrictive Prescription

a. *General*—Subject to the coinsurance amount, payment would be limited to the lowest of the pharmacy's actual charge, the 90th percentile of pharmacy charges, or the sum of the average wholesale price (AWP) for the drug dispensed, plus an administrative allowance. The 90th-percentile limit would not apply until 1992 and would be based on pharmacy charges from the second preceding payment period.

b. *Survey*—HHS would conduct a biannual survey of direct sellers, wholesalers, or pharmacists to determine the applicable wholesale price (excluding discounts). For drugs covered during 1990, for low volume drugs, and in other appropriate circumstances, HHS could rely on published sources instead of a survey. Participating pharmacies would be required to take part in the survey.

c. *Restrictive Prescriptions*—A multiple-source drug would be considered to be subject to a restrictive prescription if the physician writes in his own handwriting on the prescription that a particular brand must be dispensed. For telephone prescriptions, within 30 days after the date of the prescription, the physician must send a written confirmation to the pharmacy that the particular brand must be dispensed.

4. Payment for Multiple-Source Drugs Not Subject to Restrictive Prescriptions

a. *General*—Subject to coinsurance, payment would be limited to the lower of the pharmacy's actual charge or the sum of the unweighted median of AWPs, plus an administrative allowance.

b. *Definition of Multiple-Source Drugs*—The term "multiple-source drug" is defined as a covered outpatient drug for which there are two or more drug products rated as therapeutically equivalent by the Food and Drug Adminstration (FDA). Specific requirements regarding pharmaceutical equivalence and bioequivalence would also apply until such time as the FDA changes its definition of therapeutic equivalence by regulation, allowing 90 days for public comment.

c. *Calculation and Update*—The median AWP for a particular multiple-source drug would be based on the AWPs for all available products rated as therapeutically equivalent by the FDA. AWPs for multiple-source drugs would be updated twice a year and would be determined either on the basis of published sources or on the basis of a survey conducted by HHS as described above.

5. Administrative Allowance

a. *General*—The administrative allowance for participating and non-participating pharmacies would be $4.50 and $2.50 respectively for 1990 and 1991. The allowances would be subsequently updated once a year based on the percent increase in the GNP deflator.

b. *Mail-Service Pharmacies*—HHS could reduce the administrative allowance for mail-service pharmacies by regulation based on differences between such pharmacies and other pharmacies with respect to operating costs and other economies.

6. Special Reports and Cost Control Authority

   a. *Reports*—Beginning June 30, 1989, HHS would be required to submit a report every six months to the House Committee on Ways and Means and Committee on Energy and Commerce and to the Senate Finance Committee. The reports would include information concerning increases in prices charged by pharmacists and manufacturers for covered outpatient drugs, and would review information regarding use of covered outpatient drugs by Medicare beneficiaries. Between October 1991, and April 1993, HHS would submit monthly reports to Congress showing outlays and receipts of the Federal Catastrophic Drug Insurance Trust Fund.

   b. *Secretarial Authority*—Based on information provided in these reports, including expenditure data from 1991, the Secretary of HHS shall, beginning in 1992, provide Congress with an annual report on the budgetary status of the Trust Fund, including recommended changes necessary to achieve the established contingency margin in the subsequent year. The Secretary would have a limited authority to implement special cost-control measures by regulation for 1993 and 1994. The authority would apply if the Secretary's May 1, 1992, or 1993, report to Congress recommends changes necessary to achieve the established reserve levels, and the Congress has not enacted these or comparable changes by January 1, 1993, or 1994. Any such regulation would be effective for one year only, and would lapse at the beginning of the next year.

   c. *Limitations*—In exercising this authority, the Secretary would be prohibited from implementing a formulary, excluding a class of drugs, changing the method for calculating the deductible, or altering coinsurance, except to set the coinsurance at the previous year's level, or next year's level, or an intermediate level.

7. Utilization and Quality Assurance

   a. *General*—HHS would be required to establish a program to identify and correct utilization and quality problems.

   b. *Standards*—In carrying out this program, the Secretary would establish prescribing standards based on accepted medical practice. The standards would be based on authoritative medical compendia, except that the Secretary could modify such standards by regulation on the basis of scientific and medical information.

8. Administration and Miscellaneous Provisions

   a. *Electronic Point-of-Sale Claims Processing*—HHS would be required to establish an electronic point-of-sale claims system by January 1, 1991. This system would track drug purchases by beneficiaries to facilitate determination of deductible status. HHS could contract with entities other than carriers to implement the electronic system and to carry out related functions.

b. *Participating Pharmacies*—A participating pharmacy must be licensed under State law, must provide counselling regarding drug use and availability of generics, and must submit information on all drug purchases by beneficiaries through the electronic system.

c. *Assignment*—Payment could be made on an assigned-claims basis only to participating pharmacies. Participating pharmacies would be required to accept assignment on all covered outpatient drugs upon receiving notice from Medicare that a beneficiary has satisfied the deductible requirement.

d. *Limitation on Charges*—Participating and nonparticipating pharmacies would be prohibited from charging Medicare beneficiaries more than they charge the general public.

e. *Supply Dispensed*—Payment would generally be limited to a 30-day supply although the Secretary could authorize payment for up to 90 days (or beyond in exceptional circumstances).

f. *Payment of HMOs*—The average adjusted per capita cost (AAPCC) for health maintenance organizations (HMOs) would be adjusted to reflect this new benefit.

g. *Prescription Drug Payment Review Commission*—A Prescription Drug Payment Review Commission would be established by January 1, 1989, to provide Congress with recommendations concerning administration of the program. The Commission would consist of 11 members appointed by the Office of Technology Assessment.

h. *Studies*—A number of studies would be required.

Provisions Relating to the Financing of Benefits

1. Supplemental and Flat Part B Premiums

    a. *Premium Structure*—The catastrophic and prescription drug benefits would be financed through the combination of a supplemental premium based on income tax liability and an additional, flat Part B premium.

    The supplemental premium would be mandatory for all Part A eligible individuals (generally, individuals age 65 or over and disabled individuals who receive Social Security benefits, other than qualified nonresidents). The supplemental premium would not be treated as a medical expense for income tax purposes.

    For 1993 revenues from the supplemental premium are estimated to provide approximately 63 percent of financing, and revenues from the flat premium, 37 percent of financing. After 1993, this mix might change to reflect limitations on the allowable increase in the supplemental premium [see (e)(iii) below].

b. *Supplemental Premium Rates*—Supplemental premium rates would be set in the statute from 1989 through 1993. Preliminary estimates by the staff of the Joint Committee on Taxation indicate that the premium rate for each $150 of Federal tax liability in each of these years would be:

	1989	*1990*	*1991*	*1992*	*1993*
Total	$22.50	$37.50	$39.00	$40.50	$42.00

After 1993, rates would be indexed according to the procedure described in (e) and (f) below.

c. *Flat-Premium Rates*—The flat premium would be set in the statute from 1989 through 1993. Premium estimates by the staff of the Congressional Budget Office indicate that the premium is not likely to exceed $4.00 per month in 1989 or $10.20 per month in 1993.

After 1993, the flat premium would be increased according to the indexing procedure described in (e) and (f) below.

d. *Social Security Hold-Harmless*—An individual's Social Security benefit would not decrease due to an increase in flat premiums.

e. *Premium Indexing—Catastrophic*

(i) *Supplemental and Flat Premiums*—After 1993, the flat and supplemental premiums would be indexed according to data on (a) program costs and premium revenues in the second and third preceding years (with an adjustment for recent trends in the consumer price index); and (b) actual shortfalls in reserves (as described at (h) below) at the end of the second preceding year.

(ii) *Cap on Increases*—The combined annual increase in the supplemental premium rates for catastrophic and drug benefits would be limited to $1.50 per $150 of tax liability.

(iii) *Revenue Shortfall*—After 1993, if the increase in the supplemental premium is limited by the $1.50 cap, then notwithstanding the 63/37-percent mix of supplemental and flat premium financing, the Secretary would increase the flat premium to replace revenue which would have been collected if the limit was not in place.

f. *Premium Indexing—Prescription Drugs*

(i) *Supplemental and Flat Premiums*—For 1994 through 1997, rates would be adjusted to maintain a reserve fund at the specified percent of program outlays (as described at (h)(ii) below) based on data from the second preceding year. For 1998 and thereafter, premium rates would be indexed according to the method used to index catastrophic benefit premiums, according to data on (a) program costs and premium revenues for the second and third preceding years (with an adjustment for recent trends in the consumer price index); and (b) actual reserve shortfalls at the end of the second preceding year.

261

(ii) *Cap on Increases*—As noted in (e)(ii) above, the combined annual increase in the supplemental premium rates for catastrophic and drug benefits would be limited to $1.50 per $150 of tax liability.

(iii) *Cost Controls*—The Secretary would be authorized to implement cost-control measures effective for one year on both January 1, 1993, and January 1, 1994.

(iv) *Revenue Shortfall*—After 1993, if the growth in the supplemental premium is limited by the $1.50 cap, then (as described at (e)(iii) above), the Secretary would increase the flat premium to replace revenue which would have been collected if the cap were not in place.

g. *Premium Indexing—Procedure*

Effective in 1993, the following procedure would be followed in setting the premium:

July 1—HHS would publish program costs and reserve funds through December of the prior year. HHS and Treasury would publish preliminary notice of premium rates for the subsequent year.

September 1—HHS and Treasury would report to Congress on the premium rates for the subsequent year. GAO would send Congress a study of HHS and Treasury notifications.

By October 5—HHS and Treasury would publish final premium rates.

h. *Reserves*:

(i) *Catastrophic*—Before 1994, premium rates would be set in the statute to achieve an estimated reserve fund of 20 percent of the current year's program outlays, phased in through December 31, 1993. After 1993, premiums would be set by Treasury and HHS to achieve a reserve fund of 20 percent of program outlays, based on data from the second preceding year.

(ii) *Prescription Drug*—Premiums would be set in the statute to establish an estimated reserve fund of 100 percent in 1991, 75 percent in 1992, and 50 percent in 1993. After 1993, premiums would be set by Treasury and HHS to achieve a reserve fund of 25 percent in 1994 and 1995, and 20 percent after 1995, based on data from the second preceding year.

i. *Maximum Supplemental Premium*—The maximum supplemental premium for the first five years would be set in the statute according to the following schedule:

1989	1990	1991	1992	1993
$800	$850	$900	$950	$1,050

After 1993, the cap would be indexed by the increase in the subsidized portion of Part B benefits (including prescription drugs) from the third

262

to the second preceding year. Drug benefit costs would be disregarded for years before 1998. The cap would be rounded to the nearest $50.

j. *Part Year Enrollees*—Enrollees who participate 6 full months or less in any calendar year would be exempt from the supplemental premium in that year, and enrollees who participate for more than 6 full months in any calendar year would be subject to the full supplemental premium for that year.

k. *Married Couples with One Enrollee*—In the case of a married couple with only one member enrolled in Medicare, the supplemental premium would be computed on the basis of half the couple's joint tax liability.

2. Drug Trust Fund and Catastrophic Account

a. *Drug Trust Fund*—A Prescription Drug Trust Fund would be established. Prescription drug benefit premiums would be transferred to the Drug Trust Fund.

b. *Catastrophic Account*—A separate account for catastrophic health benefits would be established in the Medicare budget. No real cash transfers to the account would be made. If the account were depleted, Medicare Part B trust fund amounts could be expanded, but the account would be debited for principal and interest owed. Portions of the supplemental premium would be transferred into the Part B Trust Fund.

A Hospital Insurance Trust Fund Catastrophic Coverage Reserve Fund would be established. Amounts equal to the payments from the Hospital Insurance Trust Fund for catastrophic benefits would be transferred to the Reserve Fund from the supplemental premium.

3. Government Retirees:

a. *Special Credit*—A special credit would be available for individuals with taxable government annuities and small amounts of social security income. The credit reflects the fact that a substantial portion of government annuities are subject to Federal income taxation, while for moderate income individuals social security income is not subject to tax.

4. Special Circumstances

a. *Monthly Premiums for Residents of U.S. Commonwealths and Territories*—For residents of U.S. commonwealths and territories, in 1989 and 1990 catastrophic premiums would be set in the statute to cover the costs of catastrophic benefits in each territory (or commonwealth). For years after 1990, the premium would be indexed to projected increases in the actuarial value of catastrophic benefits in the United States. A prescription drug premium would be set in the statute to cover the costs of the prescription drug benefits in each territory (or commonwealth) for 1990 and 1991; the premium would thereafter be indexed to the projected increase in the actuarial value of the prescription drug benefit in the United States.

b. *Monthly Premiums for Individuals enrolled under Part B but not entitled to Benefits under Part A*—For individuals enrolled in Part B but not entitled to Part A benefits under Medicare, the catastrophic premium would be set in the statute for 1990 based on the cost of the Part B catastrophic benefit, and adjusted thereafter to increases in the projected actuarial value of the Part B catastrophic benefit.

The prescription drug portion of the premium would be set in the statute for 1990 and 1991, and thereafter adjusted to the projected increase in the actuarial value of the prescription drug benefit.

Other Provisions

1. Notice to Medicare Beneficiaries

   a. *Mailing of Notice*—The Secretary of HHS would be required to prepare an annual notice to be sent to all Medicare beneficiaries which would provide a simple, clear explanation of Medicare benefits, coinsurance and deductibles. This notice would also include an explanation of the limits of the Medicare and Medicaid programs with regard to long-term-care benefits.

   b. *Notice Concerning Participating Physicians*—A special notice would be included on the explanation of medical benefits for unassigned claims. The notice would contain information concerning assignment and participation. In addition, a booklet would be sent to Medicare beneficiaries once a year with information concerning the participating physician program.

2. Benefits Counseling Demonstration

   a. *Demonstration*—The Secretary of HHS would be required to establish a three-year demonstration project through an agreement with a private or public nonprofit agency or organization for the purpose of training volunteers. The volunteers would provide counseling to elderly individuals about eligibility for Medicare and Medicaid and assist in preparing documents that may be required to receive such benefits.

3. Case Management Demonstration

   a. *Demonstration*—The Secretary of HHS would be required to establish four demonstration projects for two years to provide case management services to Medicare beneficiaries with selected high-cost illnesses. At least one demonstration would be conducted by a PRO. Two million dollars would be authorized in each of two years for administrative costs.

4. Certification of Medicare Supplemental Health Insurance Policies

   a. *Establishment of New Medigap Standards*—If the National Association of Insurance Commissioners (NAIC) revises the existing model standards within 90 days after enactment, the new NAIC standards would be the standards for certification. If the NAIC does not amend the standards within 90 days the Secretary would be required to issue Federal Model standards within 60 days of enactment.

b. *Required Mailing of Notice*—Companies that issue Medicare supplemental policies in effect on January 1, 1989, would be required by January 31, 1989, on a one-time basis, to send a letter to their policy holders who are entitled to Medicare, explaining the improved benefits contained in the catastrophic legislation passed by the Congress, and how these improvements will affect the benefits contained in the policies and the cost of the premium.

The Secretary would be required to inform Medicare beneficiaries about current laws prohibiting marketing abuses and the way to report them, and to allow beneficiaries to use a toll-free number to report suspected violations.

c. *Required Submission of Advertising*—Companies that issue Medicare supplemental policies would be required to submit their advertising files to the State Insurance Commission for review as to whether their marketing practices comply with State law with respect to advertising used on or after January 1, 1989. There is no Federal requirement for State review.

d. *Transition for Current Policies*—If by January 1, 1989, a State does not adopt either the NAIC model transition regulation, or the new model minimum standards, policies which are otherwise in compliance with existing Medical Supplemental Insurance policy standards would be deemed to conform to the benefit changes in the catastrophic legislation, if they gave appropriate notice to their policyholders and filed for appropriate coverage and premium adjustments with the State.

e. *Free-Look Period*—Would require a uniform 30-day free-look period for all Medigap policies.

f. *Reporting Loss Ratios*—Insurers would have to report actual loss ratios.

5. Maintenance-of-Effort

a. *Employer Obligation*—Any employer who provides health benefits to an employee or retired former employee (other than Federal employees or retired Federal employees) that duplicate at least 50 percent of new or improved Part A and Part B health benefits provided under the Catastrophic legislation on the date of enactment, would be required to: (1) provide additional benefits to the employee or retired former employee that are at least equal in value to the duplicative benefits; or (2) refund to the employee or retired former employee an amount described in (b) below. The Secretary of HHS would be required to provide guidelines to employers to assist them in determining whether or not they met the 50-percent rule.

b. *Employer Option on Refund*—In providing a refund, an employer would have the option of using the average actuarial values promulgated by the Secretary of HHS or the employer's own present value of the duplicative benefits based on the Secretary's guidelines.

c. *Effective Period*—The provision would be effective for the later of two years or the expiration of the collective bargaining agreement. Employers would be required to rebate the duplicative Part A benefits in 1989 and the duplicative Part B benefits in 1990.

6. Long-Term Care Research:

a. *Long-Term-Care Research*—The Secretary of HHS would be authorized to support research on long-term care for each of the next five years. The research would focus on issues of delivering and financing of long-term care services. Five-million dollars each year would be authorized.

7. Study of Adult Day Care Services:

a. *Study*—The Secretary of HHS would be required to study adult day care services and report to Congress within one year after enactment.

8. Commission on Comprehensive Health Care

a. *Establishment of Commission*—A commission would be established to study and recommend to Congress ways to finance comprehensive long-term care, comprehensive health-care services for the elderly and disabled and comprehensive health care services for all individuals. The Commission would submit a report on long-term care services for the elderly and disabled no later than six months after enactment. It would also submit a report on comprehensive health care services for all Americans no later than one year after enactment.

9. Provisions Relating to Federal Retirees

a. *Study on Offering Medicare Supplemental Plans to Federal Medicare Eligibles*—The Director of the Office of Personnel Management (OPM) would be required to conduct a study regarding changes to the Federal Employee Health Benefit Plan (FEHBP) that may be required to incorporate plans designed specifically for Medicare-eligible individuals.

b. *Rate Reduction for Medicare-Eligible Federal Employees*—The Director of OPM would be required to reduce the rates charged to Medicare-eligible individuals participating in FEHBP plans.

10. Other Provisions:

a. *Protection of Medicare Beneficiaries Enrolled in Risk-Sharing Contracts*—Civil monetary penalties and intermediate sanctions against HMOs/CMPs would be increased for certain practices.

b. *Repeal of Authority to Administer Proficiency Examinations*—Section 1123 of the Social Security Act would be repealed, effective October

1, 1987. This does not affect the qualifications of individuals to perform their duties and responsibilities who were certified by reason of previous adminstered exams.

c. *Advisory Committee on Medicare Home-Health Claims*—The HCFA administrator would be required to appoint an 11-member advisory committee. The committee would be required to study the reasons for the increase in home-health claims denials and to report its findings and recommendations to Congress one year after enactment.

d. *Authority for Secretary*—The Secretary of HHS would have authority to take action against entities which use the emblem or name of social security programs in a manner that they knew or should have known would convey a false impression of official authorization. Violations would be subject to civil monetary penalties.

e. *Technical Amendments*—Various technical and minor amendments to the Omnibus Budget Reconciliation Act (OBRA) of 1987 and Title XVIII of the Social Security Act would clarify the statutory authority for the Medicare program.

Provisions Relating to Medicaid

1. Medicaid Buy-In of Premiums and Cost-sharing for Poor Medicare Beneficiaries

    a. *Phasing in Buy-In Coverage*—State Medicaid programs would be required, on a phased-in basis, to pay the Medicare premiums, deductibles, and coinsurance for elderly and disabled individuals with incomes below the Federal poverty level ($5700 per year for an individual in 1988) and resources at or below twice the standard under the Supplemental Security Income (SSI) program ($3800 in 1988).

    With respect to all but 5 States, this requirement would be phased in over the next four years as follows: effective January 1, 1989, individuals with incomes at or below 85 percent of poverty; effective January 1, 1990, at or below 90 percent of poverty; effective January 1, 1991, at or below 95 percent of poverty; and effective January 1, 1992, at or below 100 percent of poverty.

    In the five States using Medicaid income standards more restrictive than those under SSI, the buy-in requirement would be phased in over the next five years, with the income threshold set at 80 percent of poverty on January 1, 1989, and increasing five-percentage points each year.

    b. *Phasing in Buy-in Coverage for Drug Benefits*—Under the conference agreement, coverage for outpatient prescription drugs would be offered to Medicare beneficiaries effective January 1, 1991, subject in the first year to a deductible of $600 and coinsurance of 50 percent. States would be required, on a phased-in basis, to pay the additional premiums, deductibles, and coinsurance amounts under this new drug

267

coverage for Medicare beneficiaries with incomes at or below the Federal poverty level and resources at or below twice the SSI standard.

States would have the option to cover the deductible by either (1) covering incurred drug charges below the Medicare deductible or (2) providing the same drug coverage as the State offers to its Medicaid beneficiaries. This requirement would be phased in on the same basis as the general buy-in requirement, described above.

    c. *Coverage of Pregnant Women and Infants*—States would be required to extend Medicaid coverage to pregnant women and infants up to age one with incomes at or below 100 percent of the Federal poverty level ($9,690 per year for a family of three in 1988). This requirement would be phased in over the next two years as follows: effective July 1, 1989, pregnant women and infants with incomes at or below 75 percent of the poverty level; effective July 1, 1990, below 100 percent of the poverty level.

2. Protection of Income and Resources of Couple for Maintenance of Community Spouse

    a. *Protection of Income*—After an institutionalized individual has established eligibility for Medicaid, States would be required to allow that an individual's spouse living in the community receive a sufficient amount of the institutionalized spouse's income each month to raise the community spouse's income to at least the following levels: effective September 30, 1989, 122 percent of the Federal poverty level for a couple (currently $786 per monthly); effective July 1, 1991, 133 percent; and effective July 1, 1992, 150 percent. The monthly protected income level for a community spouse could not exceed $1,500, except where a higher level is determined necessary by fair hearing or court order.

    b. *Protection of Resources*—Effective September 30, 1989, in determining eligibility for Medicaid coverage for an institutionalized individual with a community spouse, States would be required to total all non-exempt resources held by either spouse and divide them equally, subject to the following minimum and maximum amounts: States would have to protect a minimum of $12,000 for the community spouse; States could raise this minimum as high as $60,000; however, the community spouse share could not exceed $60,000, except where a higher amount is provided under a fair hearing or a court order.

    c. *Transfer of Assets*—Effective with respect to transfers occurring on or after July 1, 1988 (or enactment, whichever is later), States would be required to determine, at the time of application for Medicaid benefits, whether an institutionalized individual has disposed of resources for less than fair market value within the past 30 months. Where such a disposal has occurred, States would have to delay eligibility for Med-·icaid benefits for a number of months equal to quotient of the uncompensated value of the assets transferred divided by the cost of nursing home care.

The current SSI transfer of assets policy would be repealed with respect to cash assistance benefits; the new Medicaid rules would apply to disposals of resources by SSI beneficiaries for purposes of eligibility for Medicaid benefits.

Minor adjustments in Medicaid effective dates may be necessary to accommodate final cost estimates.

Index

legislation, 3, 9-10, 59-60, 185

state programs, 27, 30-31, 35

Children and catastrophic costs, 54

COBRA *see* Consolidated Omnibus Budget Reconciliation Act of 1985

Commission on Long-Term Care, 164-165

Community programs
long-term care and, 76-77, 82, 111-112, 191

Connecticut Commission on Private and Public Responsibilities for Financing Long Term Care for the Elderly
recommendations, 154-156

Consolidated Omnibus Budget Reconciliation Act of 1985 (COBRA), 112-113

Continuing care retirement centers, 121-122, 200-201

E

Employee benefits *see also under* Long-term care insurance
employer entitlement liabilities, 203-204, 211-212, 212-213
Harvard retirement benefits, 161-172
insurance/entitlement trade-offs, 159-160, 172
reasons for, 160-161

Employers
long-term care and, 7-8, 14-15, 16-17, 85-86, 176-181, 197

F

Family *see under* Long-term care

H

Harvard University
retirement benefits, 161-172

—health, 163-164
—income, 162, 168-172
—long-term care, 164-168

Health care
access to, 91-92

Health care expenditures
age and, 101-102

Health insurance *see also* Catastrophic health care insurance; Long-term care insurance coverage, 32, 52, 74, 95-96, 100-101, 112-113

Health Insurance Association of America (HIAA)
long-term care projects, 179

Health maintenance organizations (HMOs)
long-term care and, 124

Home care *see also* Community programs
insurance coverage, 52
legislation, 9
nursing homes and, 237-239
quality, 229
value, 235-236

Home equity
financing long-term care, 126

I

IBM Elder Care Program, 7

Indigent care, 32

Individual medical accounts
financing long-term care, 124-125

John Hancock
group long-term care policy, 15, 17, 85, 208

L

Legislation *see specific topic*

Life insurance
financing long-term care, 125

Long-term care *see also* Long-

272

term care insurance; Nursing
homes
 as catastrophic cost, 60-61,
  220
 as presidential campaign issue, 10-11
 as public policy issue, 4-5,
  151-152, 221-222
 Connecticut Commission financing recommendations,
  154-156
 costs, 60-61, 217-218, 231-
  232
 coverage under catastrophic
  programs, 32
 definition, 4
 delivery, 64-65, 76-77, 82,
  123-124, 219, 221
 effects of increased longevity, 206
 families and, 4, 13-14, 75,
  150, 235-238
 in Canada, 77
 legislation, 9-10
 —NAIC model legislation,
  179
 need for, 4, 32, 63, 109-112,
  114, 165, 217
 —nonelderly, 77-78, 110-111,
  129
 provider groups, 5
 public awareness of issue, 6,
  14-15, 141, 179, 196
 rural issues, 17-18
 survey results, 5-6, 7-8, 63-64
Long-term care insurance *see*
also Long-term care
 as employee benefit, 8, 14-
  15, 17, 85-86, 123, 165-167,
  180-181, 208-209
 —advantages, 176-177
 —obstacles, 177-179, 205
 Connecticut Commission financing recommendations,
  154-156
 legislation, 9-10

life care at home program,
 200-201
private financing, 61-62, 75-
 76, 78-79, 80-81, 110(n),
 133-134, 189-190, 222-223,
 232-233
—design issues, 165-168,
 185-188, 199
—economic policy oriented
 approaches, 124-126
—health-policy initiatives,
 120-124
premiums, 61, 76
public financing proposals,
 64-71, 80-81, 83-85, 189,
 190-193, 201-202, 204-205,
 210-211, 221-222
state involvement, 139-141,
 142, 153-156, 199-200

M

Medicaid
 AIDS victims and, 55
 attitudes toward, 227
 catastrophic coverage, 32,
  99-100
 long-term care services, 135-
  137, 150-151, 152, 199
 spousal protection legislation, 34, 76
Medicare *see also* Medicare Catastrophic Coverage Act of 1988
 AIDS victims and, 55
 balance billing, 60, 73-74,
  79-80, 82-83
 catastrophic coverage, 3, 9-
  10, 98-99
 long-term care, 228-229
 physician reimbursement,
  60, 74-75, 79-80, 82-83
 supplemental insurance, 81
Medicare Catastrophic Coverage
 Act of 1988, 3, 9, 34, 59-60, 81,
 129, 138(n), 145, 147, 151-152,
 183(n) 185, 227(n), 253, *see also*

Catastrophic health care insurance

N

NAIC *see* National Association of Insurance Commissioners
National Association of Insurance Commissioners (NAIC)
    model long-term care legislation, 179
Northwestern National Life Insurance
    retirement planning projects, 125-126
Nursing homes
    costs, 60-61, 109, 130, 152, 218-219
    home care and, 237-238
    insurance coverage, 52
    length of stays, 137-138
    need for, 110-111, 114
    utilization, 186, 190-191

O

Older Women's League
    long-term care social insurance proposal, 64-71

R

Robert Wood Johnson Foundation
    long-term care projects, 199-200

S

Social health maintenance organizations (S/HMOs)
    long-term care and, 124
Social Security
    AIDS victims and, 55

T

Tax incentives
    for long-term care, 9, 124, 140-141, 154, 179, 202-203
Teachers Insurance and Annuity Association/College Retirement Equities Fund (TIAA/CREF)
    group long-term care policy, 180
Travelers Insurance Companies
    group long-term care policy, 123, 180
    long-term care survey, 7-8

V

Villers Foundation
    long-term care social insurance proposal, 64-71
    long-term care survey, 5-6, 63-64

W

Washington Business Group on Health
    long-term care survey, 7-8